Lecture Notes in Computer Science 7915

Commenced Publication in 1973
Founding and Former Series Editors:
Gerhard Goos, Juris Hartmanis, and Jan van Leeuwen

T0202571

Dean Barratt   Stéphane Cotin
Gabor Fichtinger   Pierre Jannin
Nassir Navab (Eds.)

Information Processing in Computer-Assisted Interventions

4th International Conference, IPCAI 2013
Heidelberg, Germany, June 26, 2013
Proceedings

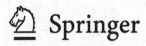 Springer

Volume Editors

Dean Barratt
University College London, London WC1E 6BT, UK
E-mail: d.barratt@ucl.ac.uk

Stéphane Cotin
INRIA, Shacra, 59650 Villeneuve d'Ascq, France
E-mail: stephane.cotin@inria.fr

Gabor Fichtinger
Queen's University, Kingston, ON K7L 3N6, Canada
E-mail: gabor@cs.queensu.ca

Pierre Jannin
Inserm/Université de Rennes 1, 35043 Rennes, France
E-mail: pierre.jannin@univ-rennes1.fr

Nassir Navab
Technische Universität München, 85748 Garching, Germany
E-mail: navab@cs.tum.edu

ISSN 0302-9743   e-ISSN 1611-3349
ISBN 978-3-642-38567-4   e-ISBN 978-3-642-38568-1
DOI 10.1007/978-3-642-38568-1
Springer Heidelberg Dordrecht London New York

Library of Congress Control Number: 2013938507

CR Subject Classification (1998): I.4, I.5, I.6, J.3, I.2.9-10, I.3

LNCS Sublibrary: SL 6 – Image Processing, Computer Vision, Pattern Recognition, and Graphics

Typesetting: Camera-ready by author, data conversion by Scientific Publishing Services, Chennai, India

Printed on acid-free paper

Springer is part of Springer Science+Business Media (www.springer.com)

Preface

Minimally invasive surgical interventions are one of the key drivers of the search for ways to use computer-based information technology to link preoperative planning with decisions and actions in the operating room. Computers, used in conjunction with advanced surgical assist devices, are influencing how procedures are currently performed. Computer-assisted intervention (CAI) systems make it possible to carry out interventions that are more precise and less invasive than conventional procedures, while recording all relevant data. This data logging, coupled with appropriate tracking of patient outcomes, is a key enabler for a new level of quantitative patient outcome assessment and treatment improvement. The goals of CAI systems are to enhance clinicians' dexterity, visual feedback, and information integration. While medical equipment is currently available to assist surgeons in specific tasks, it is the synergy between these capabilities that gives rise to new paradigms.

The Information Processing and Computer-Assisted Intervention (IPCAI) Conference was created as a forum for presenting the latest developments in CAI. The main technological focus is on patient-specific modeling and its use in interventions, image-guided and robotic surgery, real-time tracking and imaging. IPCAI seeks papers that are particularly relevant to CAI, works that present novel technical concepts, clinical needs and applications, as well as hardware, software, and systems and their validation.

The annual IPCAI conference series began in Geneva, Switzerland in 2010, followed by Berlin, Germany, in 2011, and Pisa, Italy, in 2012. This volume contains the proceedings of the 4th IPCAI Conference that took place on June 26, 2013, in Heidelberg, Germany. This year, we received 20 full-paper submissions from seven different countries. These submissions were reviewed by a total of 30 external reviewers, coordinated by the Program Committee members. A "primary" and a "secondary" Program Committee member were assigned to each paper, and each paper received at least three external reviews. Finally, an independent body of six Program Board members: Hawkes, Mori, Salcudean, Szekely, Taylor, Yang discussed all papers and a final decision was made, after which 11 high-quality papers were accepted. The final submissions were re-reviewed by the Program Committee members to ensure that all reviewers' comments were addressed.

We would like to take this opportunity to thank our Program Committee members: Ichiro Sakuma, University of Tokyo, Japan; Philippe Poignet, LIRMM, France, Thomas Lango, SINTEF, Norway; Stéphane Nicolau, IRCAD, France; Ziv Yaniv, Children's National Medical Center, USA, and Purang Abolmaesumi, University of British Columbia, Canada; and Program Board Members: David Hawkes, University College London, UK; Kensaku Mori, Nagoya, Japan; Tim Salcudean, University of British Columbia, Canada; Gabor Szekely, ETH

Zurich, Switzerland; Russell Taylor, The Johns Hopkins University, USA, and Guang-Zhong Yang, Imperial College London, UK. We would also like to thank all the authors who submitted their papers to IPCAI and acknowledge all the reviewers for their involvement and timely feedback: Louis Collins, Aron Fenster, Ren Hui Gong, Mingxing Hu, Leo Joskowicz, Peter Kazanzides, Alexandre Krupa, Andras Lasso, Hongen Liao, Marius George Linguraru, Cristian Linte, Ken Masamune, Daniel Mirota, Terry Peters, Ingerid Reinertsen, Maryam Rettman, Rogerio Richa, Robert Rohling, Tim Salcudean, Amber Simpson, Danail Stoyanov, Takashi Suzuki, Jocelyne Troccaz, Tamas Ungi, Theo van Walsum, Kirby Vosburgh, Lejing Wang, Aaron Ward, Andrew Wiles, and Guoyan Zheng.

Dean Barratt
Stéphane Cotin
Gabor Fichtinger

Organization

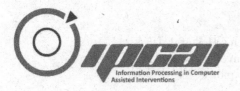

Information Processing in Computer
Assisted Interventions

2013 Executive Committee

Program Chairs

Dean Barratt — Centre for Medical Image Computing,
University College London, UK

Stéphane Cotin — INRIA, France

Gabor Fichtinger — Queen's University, Canada

General Chairs

Pierre Jannin — INSERM, Rennes, France

Nassir Navab — Computer Aided Medical Procedures/
Technische Universität München, Germany

Area Chairs

Purang Abolmaesumi — The University of British Columbia, Canada

Thomas Langø — SINTEF, Norway

Stephane Nicolau — IRCAD, France

Philippe Poignet — LIRMM, France

Ichiro Sakuma — University of Tokyo, Japan

Ziv Yaniv — Georgetown, USA

Program Board

Dave Hawkes — University College London, UK

Kensaku Mori — Nagoya University, Japan

Tim Salcudean — The University of British Columbia, Canada

Russell Taylor — The Johns Hopkins University, USA

Local Organization Chairs

Razvan Ionasec	SCR, Germany
Lena Meier-Hein	DKFZ, Germany
Franziska Schweikert	CARS office, Germany
Ralf Stauder	TUM, Germany

IPCAI Steering Committee

Kevin Cleary	DC Children's Hospital, USA
Gabor Fichtinger	Queen's University, Canada
Makoto Hashizume	Fukuoka, Japan
Dave Hawkes	UCL, UK
Pierre Jannin	INSERM, Rennes, France
Leo Joskowicz	Hebrew University, Israel
Ron Kikinis	Boston, USA
Heinz Lemke	Leipzig, Germany
Kensaku Mori	Nagoya University, Japan
Nassir Navab	CAMP/TUM, Germany
Terry Peters	London, Canada
Ichiro Sakuma	University of Tokyo, Japan
Tim Salcudean	UBC, Canada
Gábor Székely	ETH, Switzerland
Russell Taylor	JHU, USA
Guang-Zhong Yang	Imperial College, UK

Reviewers

Purang Abolmaesumi	Cristian Linte	Danail Stoyanov
Louis Collins	Ken Masamune	Takashi Suzuki
Aron Fenster	Daniel Mirota	Jocelyne Troccaz
Ren Hui Gong	Stephane Nicolau	Tamas Ungi
Mingxing Hu	Terry Peters	Theo van Walsum
Leo Joskowicz	Philippe Poignet	Kirby Vosburgh
Peter Kazanzides	Ingerid Reinertsen	Lejing Wang
Alexandre Krupa	Maryam Rettman	Aaron Ward
Thomas Lango	Rogerio Richa	Andrew Wiles
Andras Lasso	Robert Rohling	Ziv Yaniv
Hongen Liao	Ichiro Sakuma	Guoyan Zheng
Marius George Linguraru	Tim Salcudean	
	Amber Simpson	

Table of Contents

Image-Guided Interventions

Development and Procedural Evaluation of Immersive Medical Simulation Environments

Patrick Wucherer[1,*], Philipp Stefan[1,*], Simon Weidert[1], Pascal Fallavollita[2], and Nassir Navab[2]

[1] Chirurgischen Klinik und Poliklinik - Innenstadt, LMU München, Germany
{patrick.wucherer,philipp.stefan,
simon.weidert}@med.uni-muenchen.de
[2] Technische Universität München, Germany
fallavol@in.tum.de, nassir.navab@tum.de

Abstract. We present a method in designing a medical simulation environment based on task and crisis analysis of the surgical workflow. The environment consists of real surgical tools and instruments that are augmented with realistic haptic feedback and VR capabilities. Inherently, we also addressed a broad spectrum of human sensory channels such as tactile, auditory and visual in real-time. Lastly, the proposed approach provides a simulation environment facilitating deliberate exposure to adverse events enabling mediation of error recovery strategies. To validate the face validity of our simulator design we chose a spinal procedure, the vertebroplasty, in which four expert surgeons were immersed in our medical simulation environment. Based on a Likert-scale questionnaire, the face validity of our simulation environment was assessed by investigating surgeon behavior and workflow response. The result of the conducted user-study corroborates our unique medical simulation concept of combining VR and human multisensory responses into surgical workflow.

1 Introduction

Medical education is still based on the *Halstedian* approach of *see one, do one, teach one* [1] or *learning by doing* [2]. This leads to the inevitable exposure of patients to inexperienced practitioners which does not correspond to one of the principal beliefs of the Hippocratic Oath: **Primum non nocere** – *first, do no harm*. Thus, novel approaches in medical education have to be formulated. One of them can undoubtedly be medical simulation-based learning. Medical simulation learning with computer-controlled equipment provides an environment for acquiring knowledge, skills and attitudes without putting patients' health at risks [3]. It offers a highly standardized environment for objective performance assessment [4]. The possibility to repeatedly practice procedures enables mediation of error recovery strategies, skill amelioration and clinical outcome optimization [5]. Further, medical experience can be gained conducting difficult procedures or even inducing complications affecting the workflow of the procedure.

---

* Equal first author contribution.

D. Barratt et al. (Eds.): IPCAI 2013, LNCS 7915, pp. 1–10, 2013.

1.1   State-of-the-Art

Simulation-based learning in health care is commonly divided into three broad areas [6]. First, standardized patients have been used to teach clinical skills. Pioneered by David Gaba, computerized mannequin simulators have been developed for training and performance assessment of anesthetists [7] and have been in use for more than two decades. Today, mannequin simulators can be connected to medical ventilators and monitoring devices, physiologically respond to drug administration, and show pathologic conditions [8].

Second, procedural simulation for surgical skill training can take a variety of forms: ranging from animal or cadaver tissue models to synthetic or virtual reality (VR) simulators [4]. In particular, the widespread adoption of minimally invasive surgery, which is synonymous to notably long learning curves, led to the development of VR simulators for arthroscopic surgery [9], endoscopy, vascular interventions, orthopedics, ophthalmology [10], and most recently neurosurgery [11]. However, surgical training still only concentrates upon the acquisition of technical skills [6].

Third, simulation has been used for team-based training in emergency medicine and anesthesia simulation to teach teams in efficient personnel management, decision making, and effective communication for crisis resource management (CRM) in complex scenarios [8].

1.2   Three Conditions for an Effective Medical Simulation Learning Environment

Many authors agree that the combination of mannequin technology and VR procedural simulators would facilitate the integration of non-technical skills into the surgical curriculum and might even achieve the largest potential of medical simulation: team assessment and training for all varieties of medical teams and in particular surgeons and anesthetists [4], [12]. To date there still exist only a few examples of cross fertilization of the above areas in team training and notably none uses a high fidelity mannequin simulator in combination with a VR simulator. Condition 1: *few, if any of the virtual reality simulations, have the capacity for the trainer to control the introduction of an adverse event to the training scenario, although this is a common occurrence in anesthesia training* [4].

Second, many failed surgeries are directly linked to the surgeon's performance. The errors made can be distinguished into: (i) latent conditions– which are inherent within the health care system e.g. time pressure, fatigue or unworkable procedures, and (ii) active failures– which are of different type e.g. procedural violation, slips, and lapses. Thus, both surgeon and operating team should have situation awareness and experience with handling critical events which can endanger the patient. Condition 2: *The introduction of critical events into medical simulation learning environments helps to diminish the impact of disruptive unexpected events on the trainees' procedural skills. This enables the trainees to handle unfamiliar and unpredictable events* [12].

Third, there is ongoing discussion about the realism of simulators. For effective medical training the immersion into the environment is required [13]. For the setup of medical learning environments the utilization of real medical equipment is necessary. Condition 3: *The learning environment should address a broad spectrum of human sensory channels such as tactile, auditory and visual channels in real-time.*

1.3   Contributions

This paper shares our experiences in designing a complete simulator prototype and provides the technological basis to determine whether an immersive medical training environment is successful. The three conditions outlined in Section 1.2 are accounted for through the following key research contributions:

1. The combination of VR surgical procedural simulator and computerized mannequin in designing novel training setups for medical education.
2. Based on user-study, the quantitative evaluation through surgical workflow and crisis simulation for proving face validity of immersive medical training environments.

2   The Key Aspects behind Our VR Surgical Procedural Simulator

2.1   Choice of a Suitable Procedure

We concentrate on vertebroplasty (Figure 1), a percutaneous image-guided minimally invasive surgery performed within orthopedic, trauma and radiology surgery rooms worldwide. Every year about 1.4 million new vertebral compression fractures due to osteoporosis occur worldwide. Today percutaneous vertebroplasty is an assorted method that treats all types of vertebral fractures [14]. The objective of vertebroplasty is to inject polymethylmethacrylate (PMMA) bone cement, under radiological image-guidance, into the collapsed vertebral body to stabilize it. However, the complication rate is markedly high and clinical adverse effects can be devastating if not treated immediately [15]. Intensive and accurate communication especially between surgeon and anesthetist is very important during the procedure to avoid such problems [16].

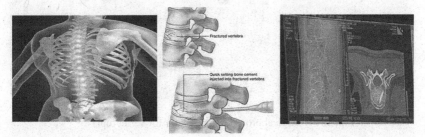

Fig. 1. Vertebrae compression requiring cement injection for stability under CT control. Images from www.healthgrades.com.

2.2   Adverse Events and Crisis Simulation

The occurrence of adverse event(s) is crucial since understanding the impact of risk or danger on clinical judgement and skill is a vital element in becoming experienced [2]. During percutaneous vertebroplasty the most common complication is cement extravasation, i.e. cement leakage. When a leakage is not recognized during the procedure, a pulmonary embolism may develop as more PMMA is injected and increasingly migrates into the venous system. A reason for a surgeon's failure to recognize cement leakage is the lack of monitoring cement flow in caudal and cranial directions during (CT) guidance. As a result, an anesthesiologist aware of the procedure-related risks is present during surgery and can interpret clinical signs of a pulmonary embolism (i.e. sudden oxygen desaturation) and communicate it to the surgeon [16].

3   The VR Surgical Procedural Simulator for Vertebroplasty

Our setup consists of a haptic device for instrument interaction (Figure 2-1), a pad into which the instruments can be inserted (Figure 2-2), a CT scanner mock-up including a positioning laser (Figure 2-3), a foot switch triggering CT image acquisition (Figure 2-4) and a monitor showing acquired CT images (Figure 2-7). A computerized mannequin simulator is placed onto the operating room (OR) table (Figure 2-5), the pad is fixed on the mannequin using a tension belt and the haptic device is attached to the table using a standard clamp. The computerized mannequin simulator is connected to the diagnostic devices (Figure 2-8) and finally draped. Real surgical instruments (Figure 2-9) can be attached to and detached from the haptic device using a clipping mechanism (Figure 2-6). CT imaging data is used to generate haptic feedback delivered to the instrument and visualize the patient's anatomy in combination with the simulated instrument on the CT monitor. The pad, essentially a box covered with synthetic skin, acts as housing for the instruments to avoid damage to the mannequin.

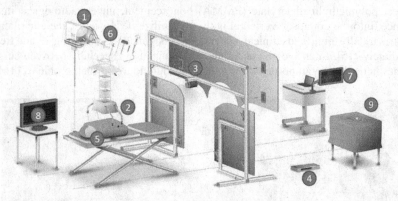

Fig. 2. VR surgical procedural simulator for vertebroplasty

3.1   Surgical Workflow Steps and Crisis Simulation

The procedural steps were extracted from live surgery video recordings and literature [17] in conjunction with the feedback from expert surgeons. Through these surgical workflow steps the aim of our simulator is to realistically represent all sub-tasks of vertebroplasty up to cement injection and successful vertebral stabilization. Table 1 describes the tasks, instruments and learning objectives within three surgical workflow steps.

Through a skin incision, the surgeon introduces a trocar into the virtual patient's body and advances it further through the pedicle into the vertebral body using CT guidance. Feedback generated by the haptic device gives the surgeon tactile information on the anatomy in contact with the instrument. Bone structures are discernible and clearly distinguishable from soft-tissue. When the desired position is obtained with the trocar inside the vertebral body, the surgeon injects bone cement using a syringe. A cement model is used to discern the amount injected and it is consequently augmented on the CT slice images. Crisis simulation: an "unexpected event" is induced in terms of a cement extravasation into a perivertebral vein causing a lung embolism. The aim here is to provoke communication between anesthesiologist and surgeon to relay proper response for this adverse event. For example, the surgeon is supposed to learn to better discern cement leakage in the CT image, before the pulmonary embolism occurs.

Table 1. Surgical workflow steps with corresponding instrumentation

Vertebroplasty			
Steps	Definition of entry point	Navigation of the trocar into the vertebra	Application of cement
Tasks	• Small incision made with scalpel	• Positioning of trocar	• Cement injection
Instruments	Scalpel	Trocar	Syringe
Learning objectives	Choice of entry point	Access path	Cement application

3.2   Technical Details on Instrumentation, Haptic Feedback and CT Simulation

Instrumentation: The instrument interface consists of a haptic device with a custom-made instrument connector and a pad, representing the patient's body, into which the instruments are inserted. The haptic device used is a Novint Falcon (Novint Technologies Inc., Albuquerque, NM, USA). It is a translation-only 3DOF variant of the delta-robot design which has the advantage of increased actuation stiffness [18]. The implications on the haptic feedback and the force reversal due to the fulcrum at the entry point are discussed in [22]. The end-effector of the Novint Falcon is detachable and can be replaced with custom attachments. Using rapid prototyping technology, we have developed an end-effector to which surgical instruments can be attached. The instruments are equipped with a plastic ball which is clipped to the end-effector socket in a ball-joint manner. To determine the amount of cement injected, we have developed a level-gauge model consisting of a level gauge with a USB interface installed in a syringe barrel (Figure 4-left). The cement injection syringe, filled with white colored water, is connected to it via a T-connector and standard syringe tubing. This T-connector makes it possible to attach the syringe to the trocar, creating the impression of injecting the cement into it, while in fact the liquid is channeled away into the measuring device.

Haptic Simulation: We use an approach similar to [21] to generate haptic feedback from CT imaging data. Specifically, two haptic primitives [23] described there, are used to generate the haptic feedback. The trocar path is modeled by a line primitive restraining the trocar from deviating. Trocar progression is controlled using a plane primitive exerting resistance as the trocar is advanced through the tissue. Instead of defining the strength of the line primitive as a function of depth, we use the radio-opacity of the penetrated tissue as an influencing factor. It is defined by accumulating samples along the instrument path, from the entry point to the tip of the instrument, that are interpreted using a transfer function (Figure 4, τ_α). A second transfer function (Figure 4, τ_β) is used to map strength to a maximum penetration speed which is enforced by the plane primitive as described in [21].The transfer functions were experimentally defined with expert surgeons. During this process, it became apparent that the bone corticalis could not be clearly perceived by the user. Therefore, we added a proxy-based surface haptics rendering method [19] reflecting the distinct shape of the cortical bone using a surface mesh derived from a segmentation of the vertebrae. This has a high simulated stiffness and we simulate bone penetration by dropping the resistance if a particular force threshold is exceeded. * *The resistance also drops in reality as the bone corticalis is penetrated and the trocar advances into the brittle trabecular bone structures.*

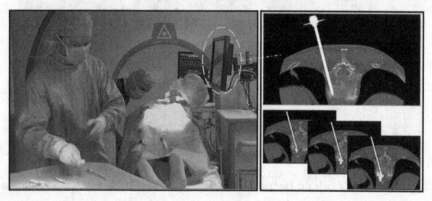

Fig. 3. (*Left*) A close-up of the operating site. (*Right*) The CT monitor shows the corresponding CT scans for (a) trocar insertion and (b) gradual cement injection.

CT Simulation: From Figure 3-right, CT imaging is used in our setup to mimic the situation in the real OR which supports the surgeon in instrument navigation, verification of access paths, and injection and control of the distribution of the bone cement. A mockup consisting of printed Styrofoam plates mounted on an aluminum frame represents the CT scanner. A line-laser fixed to the frame marks the image acquisition plane on the patient and the instrument. It can be used to define an entry point and to check whether the instrument is in-plane. Using a footswitch, the operating surgeon acquires CT images, which are displayed on a monitor placed on the opposite side of the patient. The monitor shows three CT slice images with the central image's acquisition plane denoted by the laser line and the left and right images cranial and caudal respectively to the central image. The CT data used in this visualization originates from an anonymized dataset acquired in an actual vertebroplasty procedure. The instrument visualization is achieved by rendering 3D models of the instruments in a clipping plane capping approach developed in [20]. This process is repeated with different anteroposterior offsets for the clipping plane, blending the resulting images to simulate a slice thickness matching that of the original CT slices. The bone cement is modeled as a jagged sphere rendered using the same approach. The final images displayed on the monitor consist of the CT slice image superimposed with the instrument slice rendering.

4   Results and Discussion

Four surgeons participated in a user-study involving the completion of the surgical workflow steps described in the previous section. The participants had varied experience: two senior experts (>150 executed vertebroplasties) and two junior experts (<150 executed vertebroplasties). Each participant was immersed individually in our VR surgical simulator in combination with a mannequin connected to the monitoring device. An independent person with knowledge of physiological responses and monitoring acted as the anesthesiologist. The surgeons were asked to give feedback using the Likert scale– a type of psychometric response and the most widely used scale in survey research. The subjects specified their level of agreement to a statement in our questionnaire. The 5-pt Likert scale format was: (1) *Strongly disagree*, (2) *Disagree*, (3) *Neither agree nor disagree*, (4) *Agree*, (5) *Strongly agree*. We assessed the face validity of the medical simulation environment, which is a subjective validation and usually used during the initial phase of test construction [4]. However the intent of the evaluation goes even beyond, trying to get answers related to obstacles hindering immersion into the simulation scenario and to disseminate these to the research community.

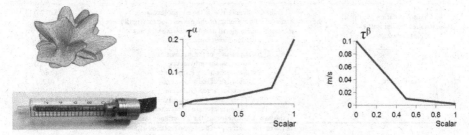

Fig. 4. (*Left*) Cement model and Level gauge with USB connector. (*Right*) Transfer functions τ_α and τ_β.

The Immersion Process: The surgeon entered the simulated operating theatre and was requested to put on medical gloves for single use. A short briefing about the patient was given: the patient's name: *'Mr. Huber'*, age: *'79'*, bone structure: *'osteoporotic bone'*, the current level: *'oxygen saturation 98%'*, and that a local anesthesia was conducted, thus the *'patient is currently awake'*. Then they were informed about the scenario and made familiar with the theatre environment. Afterwards, the independent anesthetist assumed his position on the other side of the CT scanner. The CT scanner and the patient monitor sound were turned on. The three surgical workflow steps were performed with real medical instruments and with the aid of VR, haptic, and multisensory feedback at specific instants of the procedure. During surgical workflow step 3, the simulation instructor introduced a visualization depicting cement extravasation into a perivertebral vein. Furthermore, the physiology of the computerized mannequin was influenced by the instructor simulating a lung embolism by gradually lowering the oxygen saturation from 98% to 80% beginning at a standardized point during the procedure. The simulation was stopped after the communication between the surgeon and the anesthetist occurred which determined their acknowledgment that an adverse event occurred.

Survey Results: Table 2 provides details on the average scores for the survey. The scores were categorized as: workflow steps face validity, crisis simulation, face validity and simulation environment. There were consistently high levels of agreement for all the questions. The group of surgeons thought that the modeling of workflow step 1 is realistic. The majority found that the realism is high during workflow step 2. They considered the simulation of workflow step 3 and 4 realistic as well. The questions pertaining to the face validity of the simulation setup were answered with an overall Likert score of 4.5– signifying that the simulation is realistic.

Table 2. The mean values of the statements scored on 5-Point Likert Scale (variance in parentheses)

Category	Statement: What do you think about the realism of ...	Score
Workflow Step I: Definition of the entry point	... the CT visualization of the needle ... making the stab incision at the entry point using a scalpel	4.75 (0.25) 4.5 (1)
Workflow Step II: Navigation of the trocar into the vertebra	... the CT visualization of the trocar ... the haptic feedback (bone distinguishable from other tissue)	4.5 (0.33) 4 (0.66)
Workflow Step III: Application of cement	... the CT visualization of the cement ... the handling of the cement injection syringe	3.75 (0.91) 3.25 (0.91)
Crisis Simulation Complication cement leakage & lung embolism	... the CT visualization of the cement leakage ... the presentation of lung embolism on the patient monitor (signals seen by anesthetist, audio signals heard also by the surgeon) ... the anesthetist communication	4.75 (0.25) 4.5 (0.33) 4 (1.33)
Face Validity	... the appearance of the instruments ... changing the instruments ... the movement of the instruments ... the function of the instruments ... the workflow representation ... the CT scanner monitor presentation ... the CT scanner interface (footswitch) ... the laser line representing the CT scanning plane	4.5 (0.33) 4.25 (0.25) 3 (0.66) 4.5 (0.33) 4.75 (0.25) 5 (0) 5 (0) 5 (0)
Simulation environment	The simulation environment is a realistic representation of a real OR. I would behave in the same way even in real life. The simulated procedure in the Simulated OR is good for training technical skills. The simulated procedure in the Simulated OR is good for training team skills.	4.75 (0.25) 4.5 (0.33) 4.62 (0.29) 4.5 (0.67)

Limitations: The lowest score was assigned during workflow step 3 related to the usage of the syringe and visualization of the cement in CT. Here, surgeons differed in response claiming that the manual pressure they had to apply on pushing the stamp of the syringe was either too low or too high. A major complaint of the surgeons was that the movement of the trocar used in workflow step 2 was not sufficiently limited by the bone tissue. After the surgeons placed the trocar inside the vertebra they could still move it laterally. This aspect does not reflect the surgeons experience with this instrument behavior during real surgeries and therefore it decreased the level of realism.

Overall Assessment: The complete simulation environment was ranked with an average Likert score greater than 4.5 when assessing all aspects of the realism of the simulation environment, specifically on whether it is suitable for the training of technical skills team training.

Synopsis: The goal for the modern learner is to arrive at the bedside of a real patient with proficiency already demonstrated in the requisite skills. In this process, the most expensive and scarce resource is the experienced clinical instructor. In this area, the synergy between computer-assistance and real medical instrumentation can make invaluable contributions by enabling focused and deliberate practice to further motivate the trainee. Thus, clinical education specialists need a customizable medical simulation environment to experiment with new learning models and training regimens.

In this paper, we outlined some key aspects that we believe should characterize a customizable simulation environment. We have designed a procedural VR simulator, in combination with mannequin technology, into an OR training and assessment environment. The simulator is capable of representing the entire surgical workflow including a medical imaging device simulation with the capacity to use patient-specific data, thus allowing the representation of a broad range of anatomical and pathological variety. Real surgical tools and instruments are augmented with realistic haptic feedback. Inherently, we also addressed a broad spectrum of human sensory channels such as tactile, auditory and visual channels in real time.

To our knowledge this is the first VR simulator with the capacity to control the introduction of adverse events or complication yielding a wide spectrum of highly adjustable crisis simulation scenarios. Moreover, this is the first study that combines a VR simulator with a computerized mannequin simulator in an OR crisis simulation scenario. Future work will involve the improvement of: (i) haptics feedback, in particular limiting the lateral movement of the trocar inside bone tissue and (ii) CT scanner being substituted with intraoperative C-arm fluoroscopy. **NOTE:** we will add (the possibility to use) fluoroscopy as a second imaging modality for guidance.

5   Conclusions

This study has demonstrated the face validity or realism of our medical training environment. Our conclusions validate the importance of incorporating surgical workflow analysis together with VR, human multisensory responses, and the inclusion of real surgical instruments when considering the design of a simulation environment for medical education. The proposed training environment for individuals can be certainly extended to training medical teams.

References

1. Rodriguez-Paz, J.M., Kennedy, M., Salas, E., Wu, A.W., Sexton, J.B., Hunt, E.A., Pronovost, P.J.: Beyond see one, do one, teach one: toward a different training paradigm. Quality Safety Health Care 18(1), S63–S68 (2009)
2. Kneebone, R.: Simulation, safety and surgery. Quality and Safety in Health Care 19(3), i47–i52 (2010)
3. Lateef, F.: Simulation-based learning: Just like the real thing. J. Emerg. Trauma Shock 3(4), S348–S352 (2010)
4. Gallagher, A.G., O'Sullivan, G.C.: Fundamentals of Surgical Simulation Principles and Practices. Springer, London (2012)

5. Grantcharov, T.P., Kristiansen, V.B., Bendix, J., Bardram, L., Rosenberg, J., Funch-Jensen, P.: Randomized clinical trial of virtual reality simulation for laparoscopic skills training. British Journal of Surgery 91(2), 146–150 (2004)
6. Aggarwal, R., Mytton, O.T., Derbrew, M., Hananel, D., Heydenburg, M., Issenberg, B., MacAulay, C., Mancini, M.E., Morimoto, T., Soper, N., Ziv, A., Reznick, R.: Training and simulation for patient safety. Quality and Safety in Health Care 19(2), i34–i43 (2010)
7. Gaba, D.M., DeAnda, A.: A comprehensive anesthesia simulation environment: re-creating the operating room for research and training. Anesthesiology 69(3), 387–394 (1988)
8. Fritz, P.Z., Gray, T., Flanagan, B.: Review of mannequin-based high-fidelity simulation in emergency medicine. Emergency Medicine Australasia 20(1), 1–9 (2008)
9. Heng, P.-A., Cheng, C.-Y., Wong, T.-T., Yangsheng, X., Chui, Y.-P., Chan, K.-M.: Virtual reality based system for training on knee arthroscopic surgery. Stud. Health. Technol. Inform. 98, S130–S136 (2004)
10. Rosen, K.R.: The history of medical simulation. Journal of Critical Care 23(2), 157–166 (2008)
11. Fargen, K.M., Siddiqui, A.H., Veznedaroglu, E., Turner, R.D., Ringer, A.J., Mocco, J.: Simulator Based Angiography Education in Neurosurgery: Results of a Pilot Educational Program. J. NeuroIntervent. Surg. 4(6), 438–441 (2011)
12. Schout, B., Hendrikx, A., Scheele, F., Bemelmans, B., Scherpbier, A.: Validation and im-plementation of surgical simulators: a critical review of present, past, and future. Surgical Endoscopy 24(3), 536–546 (2010)
13. Rodgers, D.L.: High-fidelity patient simulation: A descriptive white paper report (2007)
14. Krueger, A., Bliemel, C., Zettl, R., Ruchholtz, S.: Management of pulmonary cement em-bolism after percutaneous vertebroplasty and kyphoplasty: a systematic review of the lite-rature. Eur. Spine. J. 18(9), 1257–1265 (2009)
15. Ploeg, W.T., Veldhuizen, A.G., The, B., Sietsma, M.S.: Percutaneous vertebroplasty as a treatment for osteoporotic vertebral compression fractures: a systematic review. European Spine Journal 15(12), 1749–1758 (2006)
16. Freitag, M., Gottschalk, A., Schuster, M., Wenk, W., Wiesner, L., Ständl, T.G.: Pulmonary embolism caused by polymethylmethacrylate during percutaneous vertebroplasty in ortho-paedic surgery. Acta Anaesthesiol Scand 50(2), S248–S251 (2006)
17. Barr, J.: Vertebroplasty and Kyphoplasty. Thieme Medical Publishers (2005)
18. Steven, M., Nick, H.: Characterization of the Novint Falcon Haptic Device for Application as a Robot Manipulator. In: ACRA Proceedings, Sydney (2009)
19. Ruspini, D.C., Kolarov, K., Khatib, O.: Haptic Interaction in Virtual Environments. In: Proc. of the IEEE-RSJ Int. Conf. on Intelligent Robots and Systems, pp. S128–S133 (1997)
20. McReynolds, T., Blythe, D., Grantham, B., Nelson, S.: Advanced graphics programming techniques using OpenGL. In: SIGGRAPH 1998 Course Notes, pp. S90–S99 (1998)
21. Pettersson, J., Palmerius, K.L., Knutsson, H., Wahlstrom, O., Tillander, B., Börga, M.: Simulation of Patient Specific Cervical Hip Fracture Surgery With a Volume Haptic Inter-face. IEEE Transactions on Biomedical Engineering 55(4), 1255–1265 (2008)
22. Ra, J.B., Kwon, S.M., Kim, J.K., Yi, J., Kim, K.H., Park, H.W., Kyung, K.-U., Kwon, D.-S., Kang, H.S., Kwon, S.T., Jiang, L., Zeng, J., Cleary, K., Mun, S.K.: Spine needle biopsy simulator using visual and force feedback. Comput. Aided Surg. 7(6), 353–363 (2002)
23. Palmerius, K.L., Gudmundsson, B., Ynnerman, A.: General proxy-based haptics for vo-lume visualization. In: Proc. World Haptics Conf., pp. 557–560 (2005)

Generation of Synthetic 4D Cardiac CT Images for Guidance of Minimally Invasive Beating Heart Interventions

Feng P. Li[1,2], Martin Rajchl[1,2], James A. White[1,3], Aashish Goela[4], and Terry M. Peters[1,2]

[1] Imaging Research Laboratories, Robarts Research Institute, London, ON
[2] Biomedical Engineering Graduate Program, Western University, London, ON
[3] Division of Cardiology, Department of Medicine, Western University, London, ON
[4] Department of Medical Imaging, Western University, London, ON

Abstract. Off-pump beating heart surgery requires a guidance system that would show both pertinent cardiac anatomy and dynamic motion both peri- and intra-operatively. Optimally, the guidance system should show high quality images and models in a cost-effective way and can be easily integrated into standard clinical workflow. However, such a goal is difficult to accomplish by a single image modality. In this paper we introduce a method of generating a synthetic 4D cardiac CT dataset using a single (static) CT, along with 4D ultrasound images. These synthetic images can be combined with intra-operative ultrasound during the surgery to provide an intuitive and effective augmented virtuality guidance system. The generation method obtains patient specific cardiac motion information by performing non-rigid registrations between pre-operative 4D ultrasound images and applies the deformation to a static CT image to deform it into a series of dynamic CT images. Validations was performed by comparing the synthetic CT images to real dynamic CT images.

Keywords: image guided intervention, augmented virtuality, beating-heart surgery, synthetic CT, non-rigid registration.

1 Introduction

Compared to conventional cardiac surgery procedures, minimally invasive beating heart interventions limit the need for thoracic trauma and remove the need to arrest the heart. [1,2] While these approaches have grown in popularity recently, they are often limited by the lack of a direct view of surgical targets and/or tools, a challenge that is compounded by potential movements of the target during the cardiac cycle. For this reason, sophisticated image-guided navigation systems are required to assist in procedural efficiency and therapeutic success.

For minimally invasive beating heart surgical procedures, the optimal navigation system would show both the pertinent cardiac anatomy and the dynamic motion of the surgical targets throughout the cardiac cycle. It should also be cost

D. Barratt et al. (Eds.): IPCAI 2013, LNCS 7915, pp. 11–20, 2013.

efficient and be easily integrated into standard workflow within the operating room. Such a goal is however difficult to accomplish successfully using a single imaging modality. For example, fluoroscopy can only provide 2D projection images and barely shows the anatomical structures. Intra-operative MRI has the capability of displaying cardiac anatomy and motion dynamically during interventions [3], but is very expensive, requires developments of novel, non-ferromagnetic tools and devices, and is unavailable in most institutions. On the other hand, intra-operative trans-esophageal ultrasound is more accessible and clinically feasible, but its field of view remains relatively restricted. Furthermore, artifacts, such as acoustic shadowing, can limit the capacity to accurately develop volumetric models. Another cardiac imaging technique, retrospectively gated CT, can provide dynamic volumetric imaging, but the temporal resolution is limited by the gantry rotation speed and radiation dose exposure can be many times that of a static scan [7]. Accordingly, no single imaging modality appears to be ideal for the provision of 4D cardiac modeling to plan and guide cardiovascular procedures.

Some previous work has suggested the use pre-operative high spatial resolution CT and intra-operative 4D ultrasound images within a navigation system [4,5], both of which are commonly used during the standard clinical workflow for cardiac interventions. However, prior work [8] has shown that registering a 4D ultrasound sequence to a single, static CT image will result in high target registration errors (TRE) at cardiac phases other than that represented by the initial CT scan, because of intra-cycle cardiac morphology changes. To overcome this problem without introducing extra radiation dose to the patient, we propose a solution that would allow a high-resolution 4D synthetic CT dataset be derived from a single 3D CT being iteratively deformed to create a dynamic 4D sequence using 4D ultrasound data as a target. These pre-operatively generated images would be employed to provide a high quality 4D anatomical context through visualization of some or all structural components spatially co-registered (and ECG-synchronized) to the patient using standard intra-operative imaging, such as 2D/3D ultrasound. With these real-time registration techniques, an augmented reality framework can be developed and integrated into navigation platforms to provide critical information to surgeons at the time of intervention.

Much work has been performed towards estimating cardiac motion in ultrasound and MRI images by using non-rigid registration [9-12], with most of the reports suggesting that the estimated motion can be used for the assessment of both cardiac motion and mechanics. In this paper, we introduce a new concept that attempts to combine the motion estimation obtained from dynamic ultrasound images with a static CT image, to generate a synthetic dynamic CT dataset. These synthetic CT images can take advantage of the higher temporal resolution of the ultrasound images upon which they are modeled. By introducing these synthetic CT images into a navigation system, we anticipate improved model-to-patient registration and more intuitive visualization of therapeutic targets for beating heart surgeries.

Validation was performed by comparing the synthetic CT images to ground truth dynamic CT images. Quantitiative metrics were obtained by computing

the Dice Similarity Coeffcients (DSC) and Root Mean Square (RMS) errors for
the entire left ventricle.

2   Methods

2.1   Overall Workflow

The suggested workflow for generating synthetic CT images and integrating the
images into clinical workflow is described below (Fig. 1). In the pre-operative
stage, a 4D synthetic CT dataset is generated based on a static CT and 4D
ultrasound images from the patient and then brought into the OR. An initial
registration is performed between a peri-operative ultrasound volume and a synthetic CT image with the same or closest cardiac phase using feature based
registration. The resulting registration transform is then used as an initialization for the intra-operative CT to ultrasound registration, and refined by image
based registration. Surgeons can choose different visualization modes, such as
direct overlay, visualization of the ultrasound image with a "window" in the CT
volume, or simply extracting critical features from the CT of US volumes and
displaying them within the ultrasound or CT volume, to provide visual linkage
between the ultrasound images, CT images, and models of instruments that may
also be needed within the scene.This paper focuses on the pre-operative stage
part.

2.2   Non-local Means Filtering for Ultrasound Images

In an effort to improve the smoothness of the deformation fields obtained from
non-rigid registrations between ultrasound images, a restoration step is first applied on the ultrasound images. However, restoration of ultrasound images is
known to be very challenging, because speckle, as an inherent charactoristic of
ultrasound images, is tissue-dependent and cannot be easily modeled. In 2009,
Coupé et al. proposed a nonlocal means based speckle filter to perform speckle
reduction and reported competitive results on both synthetic and patient data
[18]. In this paper, we used this method to smooth the ultrasound images before
the non-rigid registration.

   The original patch-based nonlocal recovery paradigm was proposed by Buades
et al. [19] The general assumption behind it is that for those points in an image
representing the same feature, similarity should not only be observed in intensities of the pixels, but also in the patterns surrounding them. Since the nonlocal
means methods compare patches around pixels instead of pixels themselves, the
computational complexity become a common drawback of those methods. To
perform such a method on a n^3 volume with a search volume size m^3 and a
patch size p^3, the computational complexity can be $O(n^3m^3p^3)$. However, since
the method described in [18] treats each voxel independently, we were able to
parallelize the method with a GPU implementation and greatly reduced the
computation time from hours to about three minutes per volume. One example
of ultrasound image, filtered using nonlocal means with search volume size 9^3
and patch size 7^3 , is shown in Fig.2

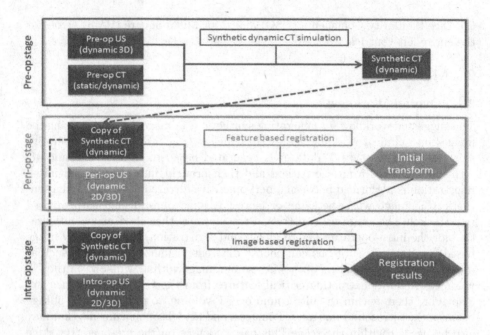

Fig. 1. Overall workflow showing how synthetic dynamic CT images are generated and integrated into a navigation system

2.3   Generating Synthetic CT Images

The methodology employed to generate the synthetic dynamic CT images is to perform non-rigid registrations between ultrasound images within a single cardiac cycle to obtain patient specific heart motion maps, in the form of deformation fields, and to apply these vector maps to CT images to provide synthetic animation.(Fig. 3) In this approach, at least one sequence of 3D TEE images, representing at least one complete cardiac cycle, and one single frame cardiac CT images must be acquired.

The procedure begins with selecting one ultrasound image, acquired at a cardiac phase close to the static CT image, as a reference. A rigid registration [8] is then performed between this image and the static CT image. This step begins with semi-automatically segmenting the inner wall of the left ventricle [20] from both the static CT image and the reference ultrasound image, and using the iterative closest point (ICP) method to align the surfaces. The alignment is then refined by a mutual information based registration [16] resulting in an optimized transform. All the other ultrasound images in the 4D sequence are then rigidly registered to the reference image as initialization for the later non-rigid transform.

After the initial rigid registration step, non-rigid registrations are performed among the 3D ultrasound images in the 4D sequence and the resulting deformation fields are recorded. This can be achieved either by registering the reference

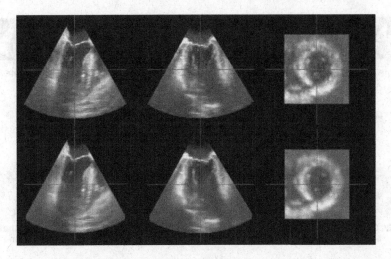

Fig. 2. An example of ultrasound images smoothed by nonlocal means based filtering. First row: original TEE image. Second row: nonlocal means smooth image. Speckle is greatly reduced, while anatomical features are mainly retained in the smoothed images.

image directly to every image in the sequence, or by performing a registration between adjacent frames. The deformation fields obtained from the non-rigid registration are used as cardiac motion maps and applied to the static CT image to generate a synthetic dynamic CT sequence. By performing the approach for each frame, we generate an entire sequence of synthetic dynamic CT images with the same temporal resolution as the dynamic ultrasound images. For this operation we employed the mult-resolution fast free-from (F3D) deformation registration method of Modat et al.[13] because of its capability of handling the morphological deformation due to cardiac motion and providing relatively smooth deformation fields.

3   Experiments and Results

Images employed in this study were acquired under a protocol approved by the institutional office of research ethics. In our validation studies, we used dynamic CT images obtained from retrospectively gated CT scans and reconstructed as ten frames per cardiac cycle as the gold standard. The first frame in the sequence is at mid-diastole. We also obtained patient-specific pre-operative transesophageal echocardiogram (TEE) images. All the data were collected retrospectively and anonymized. The voxel spacing of the dynamic CT and ultrasound images are about $0.4 \times 0.4 \times 1.3(mm)$ and $0.8 \times 0.8 \times 0.7(mm)$ respectively. CT images were acquired on a GE Lightspeed 7-VCT scanner and the ultrasound images on a Philips iE33 X7-2t TEE probe.

The first CT frame was chosen as the reference image from which the synthetic dynamic image set was constructed. Fig. 4 shows two slices, one at end diastole and the other at end-systole, from the synthetic CT dataset. After computing

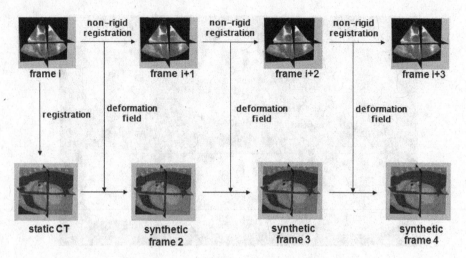

Fig. 3. Flowchart depicting the generation of synthetic CT images

Table 1. DSC between synthetic and original CT images

# of frames	2	3	4	5	6	7	8	9	10	mean
Patient 1	0.85	0.84	0.76	0.80	0.84	0.86	0.86	0.87	0.89	0.84
Patient 2	0.82	0.79	0.74	0.76	0.77	0.86	0.90	0.89	0.90	0.83
Patient 3	0.88	0.83	0.83	0.78	0.78	0.77	0.82	0.87	0.85	0.82
Patient 4	0.91	0.83	0.83	0.84	0.82	0.88	0.86	0.85	0.88	0.86
Patient 5	0.85	0.78	0.69	0.68	0.79	0.79	0.74	0.78	0.83	0.77

the synthetic CT dataset, we compared the corresponding frames to the original dynamic CT volumes. Since synthetic and original CT images have different frame rates, for each original CT image, we manually select the synthetic CT images with the closest cardiac phase to the original CT for comparison. The left ventricules were segmented from both the synthetic and original images. Fig. 5 shows an example of the segmented left ventricles from original and synthetic CT images.

Dice similarity coefficients (DSC) were computed to exam the overlap between the synthetic and original left ventricles, while mean RMSE of the ventricle surfaces were computed to exam the physical distances between them. The results are listed in Table 1 and Table 2.

We also computed short-axis slicewise DSC from basal to apical to obtain an error map along the longitudinal axis. The best and worst cases, i.e. patient 4 and patient 5, from the current validation are shown in Fig. 6, in which we observe that, for most of the frames, the slicewise DSC slightly changed along the longitudinal axis. However, we also noticed that for patient 5, the slicewise DSC for two systolic frames decreased significantly when approaching the apex. By visualizing and comparing the boundaries of the left ventricles from two slices,

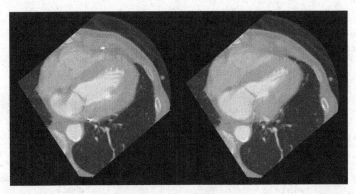

Fig. 4. An example of synthetic CT images. Left: a slice from an end-diastole frame. Right: the corresponding slice from an end-systole frame.

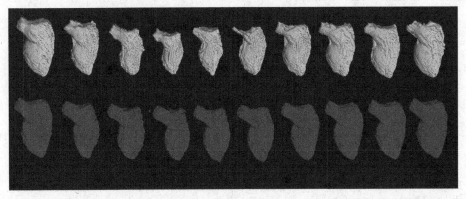

Fig. 5. An example of surfaces of the manually segmented left ventricles from original and synthetic CT images, showing the contraction and dilation within one cardiac cycle. First row: surfaces from original dynamic CTimages. Second row: surfaces from synthetic CT images.

Table 2. RMSE between synthetic and original CT images (mm)

# of frames	2	3	4	5	6	7	8	9	10	mean
Patient 1	3.06	3.10	4.61	3.69	2.95	2.72	2.79	2.74	2.75	3.16
Patient 2	3.20	3.81	4.80	4.42	4.20	2.48	2.10	2.27	2.29	3.29
Patient 3	2.55	3.11	2.72	3.91	4.09	4.36	3.42	2.64	2.71	3.28
Patient 4	1.77	3.20	2.80	2.64	3.04	2.20	2.77	2.85	2.31	2.62
Patient 5	1.83	2.35	3.44	3.50	2.13	1.96	2.47	2.44	2.04	2.46

one close to mitral valve plane, the other close to apex, from patient 5 (Fig. 7), we can see that the boundaries aligned very well in the basal slice, while the boundary of the original CT was completely contained by the one of synthetic CT in the apical slice. This implied that the synthetic CT under-estimate the ventricle contraction for this patient. The reason of this is discussed in the next section.

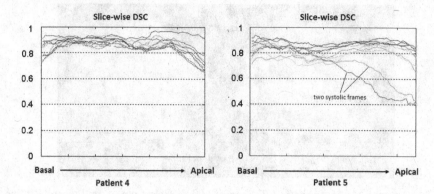

Fig. 6. Slice-by-slice dice metrics along the longitudinal axis (Each colored line represents a different cardiac frame)

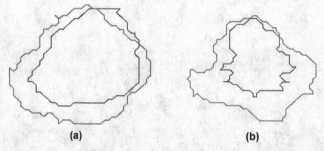

Fig. 7. Comparison of LV boundaries of synthetic and original CT image from two slices. The boundary from the synthetic CT is shown as a red curve, while the one from the original CT is shown in blue. (a) A basal slice, in which the boundaries align with each other quite well. (b) An apical slice, in which the boundary from the synthetic is much larger and contained the one from the original CT completely.

4   Discussion

The validation based on DSC and RMSE showed good results for most of the frames in a single cardiac phase, while there were some issues with two systole frames of patient 5. In the slice-by-slice DSC diagram (Fig. 7), we can see that the DSC remained high at the upper half of the ventricle for all the frames. However, two systolic frames presented low DSC at the lower half of the ventricle. Looking at these data more carefully, it became evident that the surfaces from the synthetic CT images were completely contained by the surfaces from the original CT images.

Temporal registration issues can be one of the reasons causing this inconsistency. The ultrasound images of patient 5 have very low frame rate, i.e. 7 frames per cardiac cycle, which is much lower the frame rate of the other dataset, i.e. 25 frames per second. The low frame rate makes it difficult to align the ultrasound and CT images temporally and a small misalignment may lead to large difference in the shape of left ventricle because of the fast myocardial motion at systole. Another reason could be the difference in cardiac motion during the CT and ultrasound scans. In the CT scans, β-blockers are commonly used to reduce the patients' heart rate, while this does not apply for ultrasound scans. Also, patients are usually under general anaesthetic during the TEE scans , while they are awake during the CT scans. However, this may promote the motivation to employ synthetic CT images, because the motion represented in the synthetic images is derived from pre-operative ultrasound, which should represent heart motion that is similar to the intra-operative ultrasound images.

Since the static CT images is deformed according to the deformation fields derived from the ultrasounds images, the field of view (FOV) of the ultrasound images can be a limitation of this method. Only those features that are presented in the ultrasound images will be deformed in the synthetic CT images. Clinicians can decide what features should be deformed and visualized for guidance purpose and perform the ultrasound scan accordingly. If the FOV of the ultrasound scan cannot cover all the required features, combining several ultrasound volumes covering different areas with some image stitching alogrithms may be a solution to overcome this limitation.

5   Conclusion and Future Work

This paper introduced a novel methodology that attempts to exploit the high temporal resolution of ultrasound imaging and high spatial resolution of CT imaging to generate a novel, high spatio-temporal resolution synthetic CT dataset. Our initial results lays the foundation for future work, validating its accuracy for modeling anatomic cardiac motion in different disease states, and validating the implementation of cardiac model development for the guidance of minimally invasive procedures within augmented reality environments.

References

[1] Dotty, D.B., Flores, J.H., Doty, J.R.: Cardiac valve operations using a partial sternotomy technique. J. Card. Surg. 15, 35–42 (2000)
[2] Vassiliades, T.A., Block, P.C., Cohn, L.H.: The clinical development of percutaneous heart valve technology. J. Thorac. Cardiovasc. Surg. 129, 970–976 (2005)
[3] McVeigh, E.R., Guttman, M.A., Kellman, P., Raval, A.A., Lederman, R.J.: Real-time interactive MRI for cardiovascular interventions. Acad. Radiol. 12, 1221–1227 (2005)
[4] Linte, C.A., Moore, J., Wedlake, C., Bainbridge, D., Guiraudon, G.M., Jones, D.L., Peters, T.M.: Inside the beating heart: An in vivo feasibility study on fusing pre- and intra-operative imaging for minimally invasive therapy. Journal of Computer Assisted Radiology and Surgery 4(2), 113–123 (2009)
[5] Linte, C.A., Moore, J., Wiles, A.D., Wedlake, C., Peters, T.M.: Virtual reality-enhanced ultrasound guidance: A novel technique for intracardiac interventions. Comput Aided Surg. 13(2), 82–94 (2008)

[6] Huang, X., Hill, N.A., Ren, J., Guiraudon, G.M., Boughner, D.R., Peters, T.M.: Dynamic 3D ultrasound and MR image registration of the beating heart. In: Duncan, J.S., Gerig, G. (eds.) MICCAI 2005. LNCS, vol. 3750, pp. 171–178. Springer, Heidelberg (2005)

[7] Shuman, W.P., Branch, K.R., May, J.M., Mitsumori, L.M., Lockhart, D.W., Dubinsky, T.J., Warren, B.H., Caldwell, J.H.: Prospective versus retrospective ECG gating for 64-detector CT of the coronary arteries: comparison of image quality and patient radiation dose. Radiology 248(2), 431–437 (2008)

[8] Li, F., Lang, P., Rajchl, M., Chen, E.C.S., Guiraudon, G., Peters, T.M.: Towards real-time 3D US-CT registration on the beating heart for guidance of minimally invasive cardiac interventions. In: Proc. SPIE, vol. 8316, p. 831615 (2012)

[9] Ledesma-Carbayo, M.J., Kybic, J., Desco, M., Santos, A., Suhling, M., Hunziker, P., Unser, M.: Spatio-temporal nonrigid registration for ultrasound cardiac motion estimation. IEEE Trans. Med. Imaging 24(9), 1113–1126 (2005)

[10] Shi, W., Zhuang, X., Wang, H., Duckett, S., Luong, D.V., Tobon-Gomez, C., Tung, K., Edwards, P.J., Rhode, K.S., Razavi, R.S., Ourselin, S., Rueckert, D.: A Comprehensive Cardiac Motion Estimation Framework Using Both Untagged and 3-D Tagged MR Images Based on Nonrigid Registration. IEEE Trans. Med. Imaging 31(6), 1263–1275 (2012)

[11] Wierzbicki, M., Drangova, M., Guiraudon, G.M., Peters, T.M.: Validation of dynamic heart models obtained using non-linear registration for virtual reality training, planning, and guidance of minimally invasive cardiac surgeries. Medical Image Analysis 8(3), 387–401 (2004)

[12] Sundara, H., Littb, H., Shen, D.: Estimating myocardial motion by 4D image warping. Journal Pattern Recognition 42(11), 2514–2526 (2009)

[13] Modat, M., Taylor, Z.A., Barnes, J., Hawkes, D.J., Fox, N.C., Ourselin, S.: Fast free-form deformation using graphics processing units. Comput. Meth. Prog. Bio. 98(3), 278–284 (2010)

[14] Peyrat, J.M., Delingette, H., Sermesant, M., Pennec, X., Xu, C., Ayache, N.: Registration of 4D time-series of cardiac images with multichannel Diffeomorphic Demons. Med. Image. Comput. Comput. Assist. Interv. 11(Pt. 2), 972–979 (2008)

[15] Vemuri, B.C., Ye, J., Chen, Y., Leonard, C.M.: Image registration via level-set motion: applications to atlas-based segmentation. Medical Image Analysis 7, 1–20 (2003)

[16] Pluim, J.P.W., Antoine Maintz, J.B., Viergever, M.A.: Mutual information based registration of medical images: a survey. IEEE Trans. Med. Imaging 22(8), 986–1004 (2003)

[17] Rogalla, P., Kloeters, C., Hein, P.A.: CT technology overview: 64-slice and beyond. Radiol. Clin. North Am. 47(1), 1–11 (2009)

[18] Coupé, P., Hellier, P., Kervrann, C., Barillot, C.: NonLocal Means-based Speckle Filtering for Ultrasound Images. IEEE Transactions on Image Processing 18(10), 2221–2229 (2009)

[19] Buades, A., Coll, B., Morel, J.M.: A review of image denoising algorithms, with a new one. Multiscale Modeling & Simulation 4(2), 490–530 (2005)

[20] Rajchl, M., Yuan, J., Ukwatta, E., Peters, T.M.: Fast interactive multi-region cardiac segmentation with linearly ordered labels. In: 9th IEEE International Symposium on Biomedical Imaging (ISBI), pp. 1409–1412 (2012)

Intra-operative Identification of the Subthalamic Nucleus Motor Zone Using Goniometers

Reuben R. Shamir[1,2,3], Renana Eitan[4], Sivan Sheffer[1,3], Odeya Marmor-Levin[1],
Dan Valsky[1], Shay Moshel[1,5,6], Adam Zaidel[2,7], Hagai Bergman[1,2,5], and Zvi Israel[3]

[1] Department of Medical Neurobiology (Physiology), Institute of Medical Research –
Israel-Canada (IMRIC), The Hebrew University-Hadassah Medical School, Jerusalem, Israel
[2] The Edmond and Lily Safra Brain Research Center (ELSC), The Hebrew Univ.,
Jerusalem, Israel
[3] Center for Functional & Restorative Neurosurgery, Department of Neurosurgery,
Hadassah-Hebrew University Medical Center, Jerusalem, Israel
[4] Department of Psychiatry, Hadassah-Hebrew University Medical Center, Jerusalem, Israel
[5] The Interdisciplinary Center for Neural Computation, The Hebrew University,
Jerusalem, Israel
[6] The Jerusalem Mental Health Center, Kfar Shaul Hospital, Jerusalem, Israel
[7] Department of Neuroscience, Baylor College of Medicine, Houston, TX, USA
shamir.ruby@gmail.com

Abstract. The current state of the art for identification of motor related neural activity during deep brain stimulation (DBS) surgery utilizes manual movements of the patient's joints while observing the recorded raw data of a single electrode. Here we describe an intra-operative method for detection of the motor territory of the subthalamic nucleus (STN) during DBS surgery. The method incorporates eight goniometers that continuously monitor and measure the angles of the wrist, elbow, knee and ankle, bilaterally. The joint movement data and microelectrode recordings from the STN are synchronized thus enabling objective intra-operative assessment of movement-related STN activity. This method is now used routinely in DBS surgery at our institute. Advantages include objective identification of motor areas, simultaneous detection of movement for all joints, detection of movement at a joint that is not under examination, shorter surgery time, and continuous monitoring of STN activity for patients with tremor.

1 Introduction

Deep brain stimulation (DBS) surgery of the subthalamic nucleus (STN) is an effective treatment for the motor symptoms of advanced Parkinson's disease (PD). Accurate localization of the STN is essential for optimal outcome of DBS treatment. Therefore, microelectrode recording (MER) is often utilized for target validation and refinement [1–8]. Typically, MER signals are observed both visually and with audio during passive movement of the patient's joints by the physician to identify motor related areas within the STN. MER has been shown to facilitate the accurate detection of the anatomical and motor-function boundaries of the STN [1–3, 9, 10].

D. Barratt et al. (Eds.): IPCAI 2013, LNCS 7915, pp. 21–29, 2013.

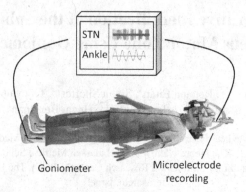

Goniometer   Microelectrode
                  recording

Fig. 1. Illustration of the goniometer setup during deep brain stimulation surgery. Eight goniometers are attached to the right and left wrist, elbow, knee and ankle of the patient and enable online synchronization of joint motion information with multiple (2-5) microelectrodes recordings.

However, passive movement is not always optimal and has some potential disadvantages. Firstly, the decision as to whether a MER response represents motor activity is entirely subjective. For example, it is not unusual that the physician is unsure whether there was an MER response to the passive movement or not; Secondly, several (2-5) parallel electrodes are usually used during surgery and it is necessary to repeat the passive movement test for each electrode separately. Finally, tremor (involuntary repetitive movement) is a common symptom of PD that provides a continuous motor activity that is not well exploited.

2   Methods

We have developed a method that aims at overcoming these limitations. The technique comprises eight goniometers that continuously measure the real time angles of the right and left wrist, elbow, knee and ankle, synchronized with STN MER of several (2-5) electrodes (Fig. 1 and Fig. 2). Custom software allows the physician to select the STN location for which a passive movement test was performed or tremor was observed during the MER (Fig. 3). The software automatically detects significant movements and allows the manual revision of the automatic selection with a user interface. Optionally, the motion can be classified into flexion/extension and average STN activity and average of movements can be plotted (Fig. 4). Finally, correlation coefficients can be computed, color coded and mapped within the STN MER trajectories (Fig. 5) to quantify the relations between the MER and joints movements. The system described has been validated and is now routinely used in DBS surgeries at our institute to assist the surgical team to identify the STN motor zones. Described in detail below are the DBS surgery, microelectrode and goniometer recordings, and our custom software.

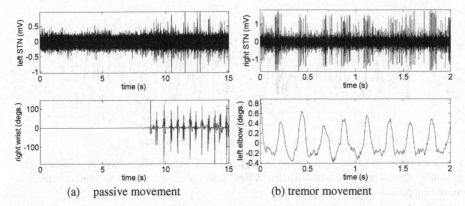

(a)   passive movement   (b) tremor movement

Fig. 2. Examples of microelecrode recordings (above) and goniometers (below) during passive movement (a) and a tremor episode (b). Different time scales are used to illustrate specific properties. (a) An increase in STN activity is observed with the onset of passive movement test. (b) The STN activity was similar in frequency and timing to that of the joint movement during tremor. Note the small angle change of tremor compared to the larger change associated with passive movement. Subjective estimation of the relation between the small and fast movements that characterize tremor is often impossible, but it can be observed with the synchronization of goniometers (b).

2.1   DBS Surgery, Goniometer and Microelectrode Recordings

Surgeries were performed using the CRW stereotactic frame (Radionics, Burlington, MA, USA). The STN target coordinates were chosen as a composite of indirect anterior commissure—posterior commissure atlas based location and direct 3T T2 magnetic resonance imaging (MRI), using Framelink 5 software (Medtronic, Minneapolis, USA). All recordings used in this study were made while the patients were awake and not under sedation. The patient's level of awareness was continuously assessed clinically, and if drowsy the patient was stimulated and awoken through conversation by a member of the surgical team. The side (right/left) of the first trajectory was chosen according to the severity of the Parkinsonian symptoms. Data were obtained off dopaminergic medications (>12 h since last medication).

MER data was acquired with the MicroGuide system (AlphaOmega Engineering, Nazareth, Israel). Neurophysiological activity was recorded via polyamide coated tungsten microelectrodes (Alpha Omega) with impedance mean±SD: 0.59±0.13 MΩ (measured at 1 kHz at the beginning of each trajectory). The signal was amplified by 10,000, band-passed from 250 to 6000 Hz, using a hardware four-pole Butterworth filter, and sampled at 48 kHz by a 12-bit A/D converter (using ±5 V input range). Local field potentials were not recorded due to constraints of electrical noise in the operating room. For both the left and right hemispheres, a microelectrode recording trajectory using two parallel microelectrodes was made, starting at 10mm above the calculated target (center of the STN as per imaging). A 'central' electrode was directed at the center of the dorsolateral STN target, and an 'anterior' electrode was

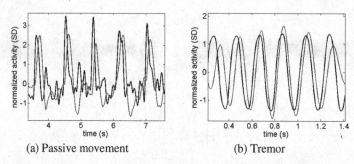

(a) Passive movement   (b) Tremor

Fig. 3. Comparison of the joint motion (black) and STN MER activity (red) in a unified scale axes after Z-score transformation. Different time scales are used to present similar number of movement periods.

advanced in parallel, 2mm anterior (ventral) to the central electrode (in the parasagittal plane). A typical trajectory was ~60° from the axial anterior commissure–posterior commissure plane and ~15° from the mid-sagittal plane. Final trajectory plans were slightly modified to avoid the cortical sulci, the ventricles and major blood vessels. The electrodes were advanced in small discrete steps of ~0.1mm within the STN along the planned trajectory. One axis of movement (flexion and extension) was recorded for each joint with a goniometer (Biometrics Ltd., Newport, UK; SG series, twin axis goniometers). The goniometer signals were amplified, sampled at 3KHz and fed into the MicroGuide acquisition system. Hence the goniometer and microelectrode recordings were synchronized (~0.02 ms accuracy) with each other (Fig. 2). Locations for which a tremor was observed during recording were marked.

Passive movement tests were performed every ~1.5mm following STN entry. A typical passive movement test included 5-10 repetitive large movements of the contra-lateral wrist, elbow, knee and ankle in frequency range of 1-2Hz. The STN entry and exit were discerned visually by the neurophysiologist as a sharp increase and decrease in the background activity, respectively. STN boundaries are confirmed and the dorsolateral oscillatory region that is associated with motor function can be automatically detected using a custom method [5]. Analysis of joint movement relative to MER can then be performed at selected STN locations and quantitative information can be analyzed. Finally, DBS was activated in the operating room for several minutes to evaluate treatment efficacy and possible adverse effects prior to implantation of the permanent stimulating macroelectrode.

2.2   Software

The raw MER signals were rectified by the 'absolute' operator to detect burst frequencies below the range of the operating room 250–6000Hz band-pass filter [11]. The rectified MER and goniometer signals were smoothed with a digital eight-order low-pass Chebyshev Type I filter and down-sampled at 200Hz. Then, the MER and goniometers signals Z-score are computed to indicate how many standard deviations

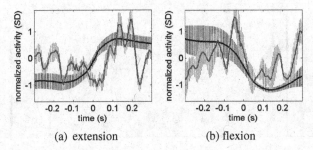

(a) extension   (b) flexion

Fig. 4. Peristimulus time histograms of average responsive MER activity (red) and average joint movement (black) during passive movements extension (a; n=12) and flexion (b; n=4). The shadows around the solid lines represent the standard error of the mean.

the MER energy and joints angle change below or above the mean activity level and to compare the physical motion with STN activity in a unified scale (Fig. 3). Pearson's correlation coefficients are then computed on these signals. The angular velocity is estimated with a numerical derivative of the goniometer signal and segments for which the angular velocity was low for more than two seconds are excluded from the MER and goniometer signals.

Time points at which velocity is locally maximal are computed and the direction (sign) of the velocity used to segment extension (positive sign) and flexion (negative sign) movements. Each segment is assigned with a unique time axis and its origin defined at the local maximal velocity point. The average MER activity and joint angle is then computed for flexion and extension with respect to the segments new time axes (Fig. 4). For an intuitive comparison of the relation of MERs to motor activity at various STN locations, the correlation values are color coded and generate a map that summarizes this information (Fig. 5). The map presents the correlation of each of the eight goniometers at all MER locations along the trajectory in the STN.

3   Results

The described method was tested on 17 PD patients. It is now routinely used in DBS surgeries at our institution and assists in validation of the STN motor zone. In addition, several interesting results have been observed using this technique. The first is that responses to passive movement are observed for multiple joints on *both* sides of the body (Fig. 5). This is somewhat surprising as according to the classical model of the STN, the motor output projects only to the contra-lateral hemibody. Mechanical coupling between joints was tested and we observed no physical coupling between joints of different limbs. Evidence for loss of specificity in the STN has previously been reported and supports these findings [12–16]. Furthermore, this may explain studies reporting bilateral improvement after unilateral STN DBS [17–19]. PD is occasionally asymmetrical, such that unilateral DBS may suffice in some cases. In addition to the reduction of surgical risk, unilateral DBS may be associated with less

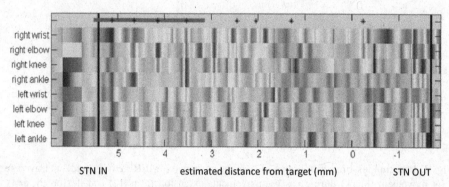

STN IN   estimated distance from target (mm)   STN OUT

Fig. 5. Correlation map of MER activity and joint angles of one trajectory in the left STN. The x-axis is the estimated distance from target defined on the MRI image (in mm). The vertical black lines indicate the STN entry and exit points. The red codes for high correlation values and blue for low ones. The plus sign at the first row indicates locations where passive movement test was performed. The continuous red line above indicates that this region of the STN was oscillatory in the beta frequency (12-30Hz) and thus expected to be associated with motor functions.

motor, cognitive and psychiatric adverse effects in comparison to bilateral treatment [20]. The second observation is that targeting the STN based on preoperative images alone without intra-operative feedback may result in suboptimal electrode location. In the case presented in Fig. 5, for example, the MER at the target of the MRI (x = 0mm) is not highly correlated with the joint movements. In this case, selecting a target 3-4mm dorsal to the one defined on the MRI may result in a better efficacy. To this end, the distribution of the motor area within the STN on 55 microelectrode trajectories of 17 PD patients was analyzed (Fig. 6). More significant correlations (p<0.05, r>0.08) are observed in the dorso-lateral region of the STN (56%; dark grey area) in comparison to the ventro-medial non-oscillatory region (42%; light grey area).

This data may be considered in the target selection of the following surgeries. For example, a consistent shift from the STN center can be computed and incorporated in the planning stage.

4   Discussion

The described method enables the surgical team to inspect the STN activity with respect to the actual movements of eight bilateral joints. In addition to the presentation of the raw data (Fig. 1), the data is smoothed, transformed into a unified scale (Fig. 2), and averaged (Fig. 3) for an intuitive inspection of the relation between the STN activity and a joint movement. A color coded correlation map enables the intuitive comparison of the relation of different STN locations to motor activity (Fig. 5). Since the goniometers and electrodes data are recorded simultaneously, there is no need to repeat the passive movement test for each electrode separately. Thus, a reduced surgery time is expected. Moreover, concurrent movements of various joints can be detected for better screening of STN activity. For example, it is possible to detect a voluntary or tremor movement of joints during a passive movement test of another joint. The method allows monitoring of STN activity during tremor movements, even though these are usually of small magnitude, fast, and may occur at several joints simultaneously. In addition, continuous monitoring affords assessment of tremor episodes that may appear frequently during the DBS surgery.

Beyond the immediate contribution to intraoperative practice, this technique may open further horizons for the treatment and understanding of Parkinson's disease. For example, a STN somatotopic map may be generated from multiple correlation maps (Fig. 5). This information may play a key role in the definition of more focal individualized target location. Furthermore, synthesized data may assist in analyzing the cause and effect between the STN activity and joints movement. This information may be useful in development of a closed loop stimulation approach [21].

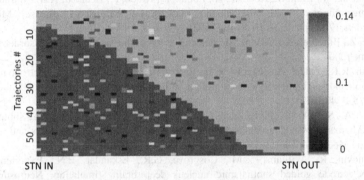

Fig. 6. The correlation of passive joint movements and STN activity along 55 trajectories within the STN. The dark area represents the dorso-lateral oscillatory region and the light grey area represents the ventro-medial non-oscillatory region. A colored pixel represents a location where a passive movement test was performed. The red codes for high correlation values and blue for low values.

5   Conclusions

We have developed an intra-operative method for detection of the motor zone in the STN during DBS surgery utilizing appendicular goniometers. This method is now routinely used in DBS surgeries at our institution and enables objective identification of motor areas, simultaneous detection of movement for all joints, detection of movement of a joint during passive movement of another joint, shorter surgery time, and continuous monitoring of STN activity for patients with tremor. Beside the immediate contribution to intraoperative practice, this method may allow a better understanding of the motor symptoms and their underlying pathology in PD. Currently we are analyzing the cause and effect in the STN-movement relationship and mapping the human STN homunculus. In addition, new methods to map not only the motor areas of the STN, but also the limbic and cognitive zones are under development.

Acknowledgements. This research was supported in part by the Post-doctoral fellowships (to RS and AZ) of the Edmond and Lily Safra Center for Brain Sciences (ELSC), the Vorst family grant (to HB) for research on Parkinson's disease, the PATH fund for research on Parkinson's disease (to ZI), and the Joint Research Grant from Hebrew University Hadassah Medical School and the Hadassah Medical Organization (to RE, ZI and HB).

References

1. Priori, A., Egidi, M., Pesenti, A., Rohr, M., Rampini, P., Locatelli, M., Tamma, F., Caputo, E., Chiesa, V., Barbieri, S.: Do intraoperative microrecordings improve subthalamic nucleus targeting in stereotactic neurosurgery for Parkinson's disease? Journal of Neurosurgical Sciences 47, 56–60 (2003)
2. Benazzouz, A., Breit, S., Koudsie, A., Pollak, P., Krack, P., Benabid, A.-L.: Intraoperative microrecordings of the subthalamic nucleus in Parkinson's disease. Movement Disorders 17(suppl. 3), S145–S149 (2002)
3. Israel, Z., Burchiel, K.J. (eds.): Microelectrode Recording in Movement Disorder Surgery. Thieme (2004)
4. Shamir, R.R., Zaidel, A., Joskowicz, L., Bergman, H., Israel, Z.: Microelectrode recording duration and spatial density constraints for automatic targeting of the subthalamic nucleus 90, 325–334 (2012)
5. Zaidel, A., Spivak, A., Shpigelman, L., Bergman, H., Israel, Z.: Delimiting subterritories of the human subthalamic nucleus by means of microelectrode recordings and a Hidden Markov Model. Movement Disorders 24, 1785–1793 (2009)
6. Amirnovin, R., Williams, Z.M., Cosgrove, G.R., Eskandar, E.N.: Experience with microelectrode guided subthalamic nucleus deep brain stimulation. Neurosurgery 58, ONS96–ONS102 (2006)
7. Sterio, D., Zonenshayn, M., Mogilner, A.Y., Rezai, A.R., Kiprovski, K., Kelly, P.J., Beric, A.: Neurophysiological refinement of subthalamic nucleus targeting. Neurosurgery 50, 58–67 (2002)
8. Montgomery, E.B.: Microelectrode targeting of the subthalamic nucleus for deep brain stimulation surgery. Movement Disorders 27, 1387–1391 (2012)
9. Temel, Y., Wilbrink, P., Duits, A., Boon, P., Tromp, S., Ackermans, L., Van Kranen-Mastenbroek, V., Weber, W., Visser-Vandewalle, V.: Single electrode and multiple electrode guided electrical stimulation of the subthalamic nucleus in advanced Parkinson's disease. Neurosurgery 61, 346–355 (2007)
10. Kim, M.S., Jung, Y.T., Sim, J.H., Kim, S.J., Kim, J.W., Burchiel, K.J.: Microelectrode recording: lead point in STN-DBS surgery. Acta Neurochirurgica 99, 37–42 (2006)
11. Moran, A., Bar-Gad, I., Bergman, H., Israel, Z.: Real-time refinement of subthalamic nucleus targeting using Bayesian decision-making on the root mean square measure. Movement Disorders 21, 1425–1431 (2006)
12. Theodosopoulos, P.V., Marks, W.J., Christine, C., Starr, P.A.: Locations of movement-related cells in the human subthalamic nucleus in Parkinson's disease. Movement Disorders 18, 791–798 (2003)
13. Abosch, A., Hutchison, W.D., Saint-Cyr, J.A., Dostrovsky, J.O., Lozano, A.M.: Movement-related neurons of the subthalamic nucleus in patients with Parkinson disease. Journal of Neurosurgery 97, 1167–1172 (2002)

14. Eusebio, A., Brown, P.: Synchronisation in the beta frequency-band–the bad boy of parkinsonism or an innocent bystander? Experimental Neurology 217, 1–3 (2009)
15. Bronfeld, M., Bar-Gad, I.: Loss of specificity in Basal Ganglia related movement disorders. Frontiers in Systems Neuroscience 5, 38 (2011)
16. Romanelli, P., Heit, G., Hill, B.C., Kraus, A., Hastie, T., Brontë-Stewart, H.M.: Microelectrode recording revealing a somatotopic body map in the subthalamic nucleus in humans with Parkinson disease. Journal of Neurosurgery 100, 611–618 (2004)
17. Slowinski, J.L., Putzke, J.D., Uitti, R.J., Lucas, J.A., Turk, M.F., Kall, B.A., Wharen, R.E.: Unilateral deep brain stimulation of the subthalamic nucleus for Parkinson disease. Journal of Neurosurgery 106, 626–632 (2007)
18. Walker, H.C., Watts, R.L., Guthrie, S., Wang, D., Guthrie, B.L.: Bilateral effects of unilateral subthalamic deep brain stimulation on Parkinson's disease at 1 year. Neurosurgery 65, 302–309 (2009)
19. Chung, S.J., Jeon, S.R., Kim, S.R., Sung, Y.H., Lee, M.C.: Bilateral effects of unilateral subthalamic nucleus deep brain stimulation in advanced Parkinson's disease. European Neurology 56, 127–132 (2006)
20. Hwynn, N., Ul Haq, I., Malaty, I.A., Resnick, A.S., Dai, Y., Foote, K.D., Fernandez, H.H., Wu, S.S., Oyama, G., Jacobson, C.E., Kim, S.K., Okun, M.S.: Effect of Deep Brain Stimulation on Parkinson's Nonmotor Symptoms following Unilateral DBS: A Pilot Study. Parkinson's Disease, 507416 (2011)
21. Rosin, B., Slovik, M., Mitelman, R., Rivlin-Etzion, M., Haber, S.N., Israel, Z., Vaadia, E., Bergman, H.: Closed-loop deep brain stimulation is superior in ameliorating parkinsonism. Neuron 72, 370–384 (2011)

Model-Guided Placement of Cerebral Ventricular Catheters

Ingerid Reinertsen[1,2,4], Asgeir Jakola[2,3,4], Ole Solheim[2,3,4],
Frank Lindseth[1,2,4], and Geirmund Unsgård[2,3,4]

[1] SINTEF Dept. Medical Technology, Trondheim, Norway
[2] Norwegian University of Science and Technology (NTNU), Trondheim, Norway
[3] Department of Neurosurgery, St. Olav University Hospital, Trondheim, Norway
[4] National Competence Services for Ultrasound and Image Guided Therapy,
St. Olav University Hospital, Trondheim, Norway
Ingerid.Reinertsen@sintef.no

Abstract. Purpose: Freehand placement of external ventricular drainage is not sufficiently accurate and precise. In the absence of high quality pre-operative 3D images, we propose the use of an average model for guidance of ventricular catheters. **Methods:** The model was segmented to extract the ventricles and registered to five normal volunteers using a combination of landmark based and surface based registration. The proposed method was validated by comparing the use of the average model to the use of volunteer-specific images. **Results:** The position and orientation of the ventricles were compared and the distances between the target points at the left and right foramen of Monroe were computed (Mean±std: 5.65±1.60mm and 6.05±1.34mm for the left and right side respectively). **Conclusions:** Although an average model for guidance of a surgical procedure has a number of limitations, our initial experiments show that the use of a model might provide sufficient guidance for determination of the angle of insertion. Future work will include further clinical testing and possible refinement of the model.

1 Introduction

Placement of ventricular catheters is one of the most common neurosurgical procedures both in the adult and in the pediatric population. By neurosurgeons it is considered a fast and uncomplicated routine procedure that is often performed in the operating room under emergency conditions or in the intensive care unit without rigid head fixation or neuronavigation systems. The standard surgical technique is a freehand pass with the catheter through a burr hole in the skull. The point of entry (Kocher's point) is located approximately 2,5 cm from the midline and 1 cm anterior to the coronal suture. The choice of trajectory to reach the lateral ventricle is based on external landmarks such as the medial canthus of the eye and the external auditory meatus. As these external landmarks are covered with surgical drapes during catheter insertion, successful placement of the catheter relies heavily on the surgeon's sense of spatial orientation. Free flow of cerebrospinal fluid (CSF) from the distal end of the catheter is considered an

D. Barratt et al. (Eds.): IPCAI 2013, LNCS 7915, pp. 30–39, 2013.

indication of satisfactory placement. Unfortunately, occlusion of the ventricular catheter due to sub-optimal placement is a major cause of re-operations and complications related to the surgical procedure. Toma et al. [1] reported that only 39.9% of the 183 ventricular catheters in their retrospective study were correctly placed within the frontal horn of the lateral ventricle. Other groups have presented similar results. Huyette et al. [2] retrospectively evaluated post-operative CT scans from 97 patients and found that only 56.1% of the catheters were in the ipsi-lateral ventricle. They also found that 22.4% of the catheters were placed in non-ventricular spaces. Even the successfully placed catheters were on average 16 mm from the target within the lateral ventricle at the foramen of Monroe. On average, two passes were needed for successful placement.

In order to reduce the high fraction of catheters incorrectly or sub-optimally placed, different image guidance techniques have been developed. Hayhust et al. [3,4] developed and evaluated a system based on an electromagnetic positioning system. They concluded that image guidance reduced poor placement of the catheter and resulted in a significant decrease in the early shunt revision rate. Levitt et al. [5] also found that the accuracy of catheter placement was significantly improved with image guidance in a retrospective study of 102 shunt surgeries in 89 patients.

Even though image guidance seems to improve the accuracy of the catheter placement, the need for additional imaging and rigid head fixation makes the solution unattractive or even unfeasible in many cases, as pointed out by Kestle [6]. In general, only a few 2D CT images of the patient are available before surgery. In this paper, we therefore investigate the use of a pre-defined model to guide the placement of ventricular catheters in the absence of patient-specific 3D images suited for traditional image guidance. The model is an adapted version of the ICBM152 non-linear symmetric average model [8,7], and can be loaded into a standard neuronavigation system. The ventricular catheter itself can be tracked either using electromagnetic tracking as suggested by Hayhurst et al. [3] or by optical tracking as suggested by Reinertsen et al. [9]. The model is then registered to the patient using a set of anatomical landmarks in addition to a a surface trajectory acquired with a tracked pointer on the patient's head. The registered model can then be used to plan the entry point and more importantly, the trajectory toward the ipsi-lateral ventrice and the foramen of Monroe.

Because there is no gold standard for the position and orientation of the ventricles, we have validated this approach on five normal volunteers. We have obtained MR images of the volunteers and compare the model to volunteer-specific data, both registered to the volunteer. The adaption of the average model and the validation experiments are detailed in the following sections.

2   Methods

2.1   Segmentation

The ICBM-152 average average brain model was segmented using the Freesurfer package, which is documented and freely available for download

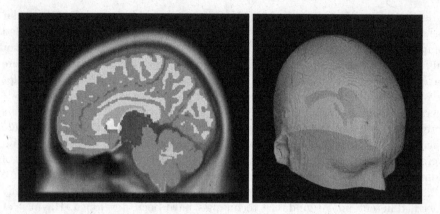

Fig. 1. Sagittal slice of the segmented model (left) and the skin surface with the segmented ventricles(right)

online (http://surfer.nmr.mgh.harvard.edu/). The automatic segmentation of brain structures is described in Fischl et al. [14,15]. Following the full brain segmentation, we extracted the labels corresponding to the left and right lateral ventricles and the third ventricle. The third ventricle is important in order to clearly see the foramen of Monroe which is the target point for the placement of ventricular catheters. We then segmented the skin surface from the model using the foreground filter that is part of 3DSlicer [16] (http://www.slicer.org/). This method uses the Otsu threshold algorithm [17] and morphological operators to achieve segmentation. The segmented model and the skin surface are shown in Figure 1.

For validation purposes, we obtained T1-weighted MR images of the five normal volunteers that participated in the study. The MR images of the volunteers were also segmented using the Freesurfer package. The ventricles were extracted from the label dataset and the skin surfaces were segmented using the foreground filter in 3DSlicer. We also manually identified seven anatomical landmarks (lateral and medial cathus of both eyes, the nasion and tragus on each side) in each image volume.

2.2   Identification of Skin Landmarks in the Average Model

The use of anatomical landmarks for model-to-patient registration requires identification of anatomical skin landmarks in the average model. When the model was generated [8,7], the optimization of the registration parameters was performed only on the brain. The skin, skull, eyes, muscles etc. were excluded from the registration algorithm using a brain mask. Consequently, the skin surface in the average model is blurry and reliable identification of anatomical skin landmarks in this volume is associated with considerable uncertainty. We therefore identified the seven anatomical landmarks in the MR images of the five volunteers. The MR images of the volunteers were then registered to the average model using the elastix software [18] built on top the InsightToolkit (ITK) [19]. In a first step, we performed a rigid body registration and then in a second step a full 12 parameters affine registration. In both steps we used the mutual information similarity measure [23] and a standard gradient descent optimization technique. The resulting transforms were then applied to the anatomical landmarks identified for the five volunteers bringing the landmarks into model space. The landmarks corresponding to each anatomical location from the five volunteers were then averaged to generate seven landmarks in stereotactic space. The fact that the skin surface in the average model is blurry obviously represents a source of uncertainty in in the segmentation of the skin surface. Therefore, we optimized the parameters of the skin surface segmentation in order to minimize the distance between the segmented surface and the anatomical landmarks. The mean distance between the points and the surface is 1.14 ± 0.53 mm.

2.3 Patient Registration

Following skin surface segmentation and identification of anatomical landmarks, registration of the model to the volunteer could be performed. In a first step, we used an optically tracked pointer (Northern Digital Inc., Waterloo, ON) to identify seven anatomical points on the volunteer. We then continuously sampled points with the tracked pointer by moving the pointer tip over the available skin surface (face and scalp). Our approach for image-to-patient registration was then to perform a landmark based registration in a first step, and a surface based registration in a second step. The landmark based registration thus provides a starting position for the surface based registration. In situations where surface points do not sufficiently cover the facial region and/or the sagittal and coronal directions, the surface based registration might not be sufficiently restrained particularly when it comes to the rotation around the axial direction. This may cause the surface based registration to converge to a local minimum instead of the correct solution. For surface based registration, we use a modified version of the ICP algorithm [20], and in order to make the algorithm more robust, the landmark based registration is included in the iteration loop. For each iteration, the landmark based transform and the surface based transform are computed separately and the final transform for a given iteration is computed using the following equation:

$$T = \frac{1}{n}T_{landmark} + (1 - \frac{1}{n})T_{surface}$$

where n is the current iteration number. The final transform T in each iteration is thus a weighted combination of (1) a rigid body transform between the automatically generated points in the image and the corresponding anatomical landmarks identified on the patient and (2) a modified version of the iterative closest point (ICP) algorithm [20] using the points sampled on the patients head and the segmented skin surface. The resulting transformation T is then applied to both the anatomical landmarks and the surface points. The use of the weighting factor $1/n$ means that the first iteration ($n=1$) gives a pure landmark based transform, which gives a reasonable starting position for the following iterations where the weight of the landmark based transform will be gradually reduced and the surface based registration will be more important. The original ICP algorithm estimates a least squares fit between the source and target point sets. The least squares solution is known to be extremely sensitive to outliers and missing data. For our application, outliers and missing data may occur if the pointer position is sampled when the pointer is not in contact with the patients skin or when the pointer is not seen by the tracking camera. To make the surface registration more robust, we incorporated the least trimmed squares (LTS) estimator [21] to reduce the influence of possible outliers. As in the original ICP algorithm, all the source points are matched to the closest target point, but a user defined percentage (LTS ratio) of the point pairs with the largest corresponding distances are excluded from the least squares computation.

3   Experiments

3.1   Data

We validated the method on five normal volunteers. The volunteers were placed in a supine position. The head was immobilized using a vacuum pillow routinely used for shunt patients. Using our in-house navigation system with a computer tracked pointer, we acquired the position of seven anatomical landmarks: lateral and medial canthus of both eyes, the nasion and tragus on each side. We finally acquired a set of surface points by continuously sampling a trajectory on the skin surface.

3.2   Registration

Using the image-to-patient registration method described in section 2.3, we retrospectively registered the average model to the volunteer. We used a seven parameters linear transformation (3 translations, 3 rotations and isotropic scaling) and a LTS ratio of 20%. The landmarks corresponding to the volunteer in question were excluded from the average point set in model space in order to avoid any bias. The resulting transformation was also applied to the segmented ventricles. In order to validate the position and orientation of the resulting ventricles, we used the T1-weighted MR image of the volunteer. We registered the volunteer-specific dataset to the volunteer in a similar manner. For this registration, we used a rigid body transformation (3 translations, 3 rotations) and a LTS ratio of 20%. An example of anatomical landmarks and surface points registered to the model and to volunteer-specific data is shown in Figure 2. The resulting transformation was finally applied to the segmented volunteer-specific ventricles. We then compared the ventricles obtained using the average model and those obtained using volunteer-specific data. The comparison between the model ventricles and the volunteer specific ventricles is shown in Figure 3. Color coded maps showing the distance between the two surfaces for each dataset are shown in Figure 4. We also identified the target points for a ventricular catheter

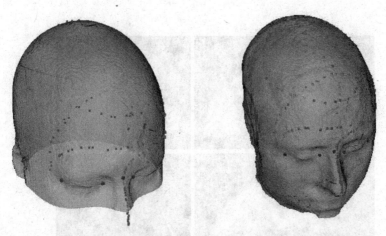

Fig. 2. Anatomical landmarks and surface trajectory registered to the model (left) and to the volunteer-specific data (right)

in each lateral ventricle immediately above the foramen of Monroe and computed the distances between the target points in the average model and the volunteer-specific datasets. The distances are presented in Table 1.

4   Results

We measured the distance between the target points in the average model and in the volunteer-specific dataset. We also investigated if the model-based targets fall inside the volunteer-specific ventricles.The results are presented in Table 1. The overlap between the ventricles segmented from the model and the ventricles segmented from the volunteer specific datasets is shown in Figure 3, and color coded maps showing the distance between the two surfaces are shown in Figure 4.

Table 1. Distances between the target points (left and right foramen of Monroe) in the average model and the volunteer-specific datasets. "Yes" or "no" indicates if the model target point in question falls inside the voluntee-specific ventricle.

Volunteer	Distance left in mm. (Inside)	Distance right in mm. (Inside)
1	4.66 (yes)	5.15 (no)
2	7.11 (yes)	6.88 (yes)
3	5.92 (no)	6.61 (yes)
4	3.42 (no)	4.19 (yes)
5	7.12 (yes)	7.42(yes)
Mean±std (mm)	5.65±1.60	6.05±1.34

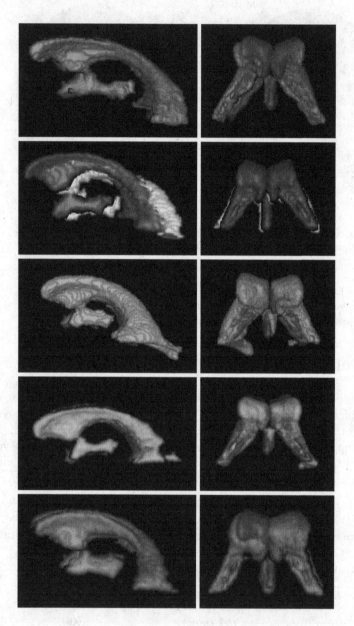

Fig. 3. Model ventricles (dark blue) compared to volunteer-specific ventricles (colors) in the frame of reference of the volunteer for the different five volunteers (rows). Each color represent one person. Sagittal view (left) and coronal view (right).

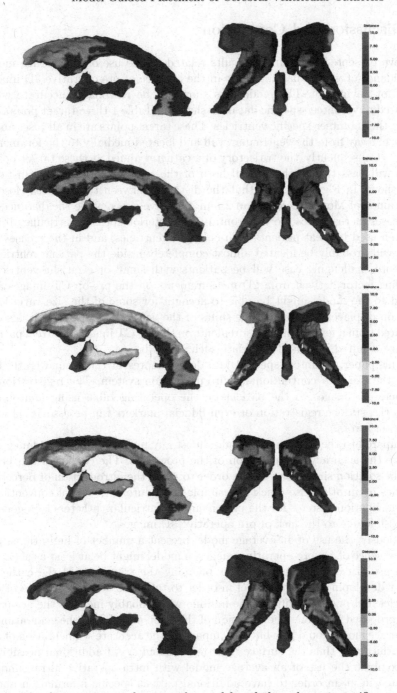

Fig. 4. The distance in mm between the model and the volunteer-specific ventricles mapped onto the model for each dataset. Negative values indicate that the model surface is inside the volunteer-specific surface, and positive values indicate that the model-surface is outside the volunteer-specific surface. All distances in mm

5   Discussion and Conclusion

We have presented preliminary results related to the use of an average model for guidance of ventricular catheters in the absence of pre-operative 3D images suited for navigation. The model has shown to be reasonably accurate when compared to volunteer-specific data. As shown in Table 1 three target points fall outside the volunteer-specific ventricles. These target points are in all cases about one voxel away from the ventricular wall and located medially to the foramen of Monroe. Consequently, the trajectory of a catheter aimed at these target points points will pass trough the frontal horn of the lateral ventricle. The distance maps shown in Figure 4 show that the distance between the surfaces close to the foramen of Monroe is less than 2 mm in all five cases, while the distances in some cases increase close to the frontal and posterior horns. Ventricular drains are often used to treat patients with enlarged ventricles, and in these cases the model will probably be located almost completely inside the patient ventricles. The more challenging case will be patients with small or even slit ventricles. A scaling factor derived from 2D measurements on the pre-op CT images and applied to the model might be able to account for some of the size variations. Common displacements or midline-shifts of the ventricles can probably also be estimated from a few simple measurements on the 2D CT images, but real patient data are required in order to validate such methods.

In this paper, volunteer-specific data do not represent the ground truth, but rather the use of a conventional neuro-navigation system. The registration of pre-operative images to the patient on the operating table using anatomical landmarks, surface registration or even fiducial markers can be associated with significant errors.

Compared to the freehand method, almost any means of image guidance will improve the accuracy and precision of the procedure. The challenge will be to keep the solution simple and fast in order to avoid the introduction of perceived obstacles in an otherwise quick and simple procedure. The use of conventional neuro-navigation systems for the placement of ventricular catheters is in general not possible due to the lack of pre-operative 3D images.

Obviously, the use of an average model present a number of limitations, but in the absence of 3D pre-operative images, a model might be at least as accurate as the use of external landmarks for planning the trajectory of the catheter. Further development of the model in order to take into account the size of the ventricles and possible shifts in the midline will probably increase the accuracy of the proposed solution. The inclusion of the scalp and skin in the generation of the average model could also have an impact on the accurate segmentation of the skin surface and thus the surface registration results. An additional possibility is to combine the use of an average model with intra-operative ultrasound as suggested in [9] in order to have additional patient specific information about the size, shape, position and orientation of the ventricles.

References

1. Toma, A.K., et al.: External Ventricular Drain Insertion Accuracy: Is There a Need for Change in Practice? Neurosurgery 65(6), 1197–1201 (2009)
2. Huyette, D.R., et al.: Accuracy of the freehand pass technique for ventriculostomy catheter placement: retrospective assessment using computer tomography scans. J. of Neurosurg. 108, 88–91 (2008)
3. Hayhurst, C., et al.: Application of electromagnetic technology to neuronavigation: a revolution in image-guided neurosurgery. J. of Neurosurg. 111, 1179–1184 (2009)
4. Hayhurst, C., et al.: Effect of electromagnetic-navigated shunt placement on failure rates: a prospective multicenter study. J. of Neurosurg. (April 2010)
5. Levitt, M.R., et al.: Image-guided cerebrospinal fluid shunting in children: catheter accuracy and shunt survival. J. of Neurosurg.: Pediatrics 10 (August 2012)
6. Kestle, J.R.W.: Editorial: Shunt malfunction. J. of Neurosurg. 113 (December 2010)
7. Fonov, V.S., et al.: Unbiased average age-appropriate atlases for pediatric studies. NeuroImage 54(1) (2011)
8. Fonov, V.S., et al.: Unbiased nonlinear average age-appropriate brain templates from birth to adulthood. NeuroImage 47(1), S102 (2009)
9. Reinertsen, I., et al.: A new system for 3D ultrasound-guided placement of cerebral ventricle catheters. IJCARS 7(1) (2012)
10. Guimond, A., et al.: Average brain models: A Convergence Study. Computer Vision and Image Understanding 77(2), 192–210 (1999)
11. Bullitt, E., et al.: Vessel tortuosity and brain tumor malignancy: A blinded study. Academic Radiology 12, 1232–1240 (2005)
12. Grabner, G., Janke, A.L., Budge, M.M., Smith, D., Pruessner, J.C., Collins, D.L.: Symmetric Atlasing and Model Based Segmentation: An Application to the Hippocampus in Older Adults. In: Larsen, R., Nielsen, M., Sporring, J., et al. (eds.) MICCAI 2006. LNCS, vol. 4191, pp. 58–66. Springer, Heidelberg (2006)
13. Collins, D.L., et al.: Automatic 3D Model-Based Neuroanatomical Segmentation. Human Brain Mapping 3, 190–208 (1995)
14. Fischl, B., et al.: Whole brain segmentation: automated labeling of neuroanatomical structures in the human brain. Neuron 33, 341–355 (2002)
15. Fischl, B., et al.: Sequence-independent segmentation of magnetic resonance images. Neuroimage 23(suppl. 1), S69–S84 (2004)
16. Pieper, S., et al.: The NA-MIC Kit: ITK, VTK, Pipelines, Grids and 3D Slicer as an Open Platform for the Medical Image Computing Community. Proceedings of IEEE From Nano to Macro 2006 1, 698–701 (2006)
17. Otsu, N.: A threshold selection method from gray-level histograms. IEEE Transactions on Systems, Man and Cybernetics 9(1), 62–66 (1979)
18. Klein, S., et al.: elastix: a toolbox for intensity-based medical image registration. IEEE Trans. Med. Imaging 29, 196–205 (2010)
19. Ibanez, L., et al.: The ITK Software Guide: The Insight Segmentation and Registration Toolkit, New York (2005)
20. Besl, P.J., McKay, N.D.: A Method for Registration of 3D Shapes. IEEE Trans. on PAMI 14, 239–256 (1992)
21. Rousseeuw, P.J., Annick, M.L.L.R.: Robust Regression and Outlier Detection (1987)

Ultrasound-Based Image Guidance for Robot-Assisted Laparoscopic Radical Prostatectomy: Initial *in-vivo* Results

Omid Mohareri[1], Caitlin Schneider[1], Troy K. Adebar[2], Mike C. Yip[3],
Peter Black[4], Christopher Y. Nguan[4], Dale Bergman[5], Jonathan Seroger[5],
Simon DiMaio[5], and Septimiu E. Salcudean[1]

[1] Department of Electrical and Computer Engineering,
University of British Columbia, Vancouver, Canada
[2] Department of Mechanical Engineering, Stanford University, CA, United States
[3] Department of Bioengineering, Stanford University, CA, United States
[4] Department of Urologic Sciences, Faculty of Medicine,
University of British Columbia, Vancouver, Canada
[5] Intuitive Surgical Inc., Sunnyvale, CA, United States

Abstract. This paper describes the initial clinical evaluation of a real-time ultrasound-based guidance system for robot-assisted laparoscopic radical prostatectomy (RALRP). The surgical procedure was performed on a live anaesthetized canine with a da Vinci SI robot. Intraoperative imaging was performed using a robotic transrectal ultrasound (TRUS) manipulator and a bi-plane TRUS transducer. Two registration methods were implemented and tested: (i)using specialized fiducials placed at the air-tissue boundary, 3D TRUS data were registered to the da Vinci stereo endoscope with an average TRE of 2.37 ± 1.06 mm, (ii)using localizations of the da Vinci manipulator tips in 3D TRUS images, 3D TRUS data were registered to the kinematic frame of the da Vinci manipulators with average TRE of 1.88 ± 0.88 mm using manual tool tip localization, and average TRE of 2.68 ± 0.98 mm using an automatic tool tip localization algorithm. Registration time was consistently less than 2 minutes when performed by two experienced surgeons after limited learning. The location of the TRUS probe was remotely controlled through part of the procedure by a da Vinci tool, with the corresponding ultrasound images being displayed on the surgeon console using TilePro. Automatic tool tracking was achieved with angular accuracy of 1.65 ± 1.24 deg. This work demonstrates, for the first time, the *in-vivo* use of a robotically controlled TRUS probe calibrated to the da Vinci robot, and will allow the da Vinci tools to be tracked for safety and to be used as pointers for regions of interest to be imaged by ultrasound.

Keywords: Image guided surgery, Robot-assisted prostate surgery, da Vinci surgical robot, 3D ultrasound.

D. Barratt et al. (Eds.): IPCAI 2013, LNCS 7915, pp. 40–50, 2013.
© Springer-Verlag Berlin Heidelberg 2013

1   Introduction

Robot-assisted laparoscopic radical prostatectomy (RALRP) using the da Vinci system (Intuitive Surgical Inc., Sunnyvale, CA) has become widely accepted and is now used to perform up to 80% of radical prostatectomy (RP) procedures in the United States [1]. While robot assistance has enhanced the visualization of the surgical site and has improved dexterity over standard laparoscopic instruments, achievement of the three main RP outcomes - cancer control, urinary control and sexual function - is still highly dependent on the expert understanding of the prostate and periprostatic anatomy [10]. It can be challenging to localize critical structures such as the bladder neck, the neuro-vascular bundles (NVB), the urethral sphincter muscle, and to define accurate dissection planes solely using visual cues [9]. Intraoperative imaging may aid the surgeons in localizing these structures. Trans-rectal ultrasound (TRUS) is the most commonly applied modality for imaging the prostate and the only approach implementable in a standard operating room (OR). To be useful, the TRUS transducer must be positioned and controlled by the surgeon in an intuitive way. Furthermore, the TRUS images should be displayed at a correct location relative to the da Vinci vision system and the da Vinci instruments.

Recently, robotic TRUS manipulators have been used for real-time guidance during RALRP procedures [10,9,8]. Hung *et al.* used a robotic TRUS manipulator (ViKY system, EndoControl medical, Grenoble, France) for real-time monitoring of the prostate and periprostatic anatomy. They showed that using robotic TRUS is feasible and safe, and it provided the surgeon with valuable anatomic information [9]. Long *et al.* used the same TRUS robot to visualize real-time bladder neck dissection, NVB release and apical dissection [10]. They showed that using robotic TRUS resulted in no positive surgical margins in five patients. Han *et al.* used their custom-made robotic TRUS manipulator for improved visualization of the NVB. This study demonstrated that the prostate can be safely scanned using the TRUS robot, to reconstruct the 3D images of the prostate gland and adjacent NVB, and the intra-abdominal da Vinci instruments can be clearly visualized in the TRUS images [8].

In previous *in-vivo* studies, the TRUS manipulators have not been registered to the da Vinci robot or camera, and therefore the ultrasound image could not be presented at the correct location in space relative to the console view or the da Vinci instruments. The control of the TRUS image location from within the da Vinci console has also not been demonstrated before in *in-vivo* studies. The work presented in this paper describes the evaluation of a robotic TRUS guidance system, performed *in-vivo* on a canine model. The contributions of this study include showing that registered robotic TRUS imaging can be deployed and used easily during surgery with high accuracy in a short time, and that TRUS imaging can be controlled in the registered coordinate system directly from within the surgeon console. We used a live anaesthetized animal before engaging in human studies in order to verify the feasibility and the safety of our approach, which requires some additional steps to conventional RALRP. The canine model is the most often used for various urologic procedures in the kidney, urethra, bladder, prostate and bowel [5].

Similarly to [2], the robotic system used in this work for real-time TRUS imaging has two degrees of freedom (translation along the TRUS axis and rotation about the TRUS axis) and is mounted on a brachytherapy stabilizer. In order to determine the location of the TRUS probe with respect to the da Vinci coordinate system, we follow the approach from [11] to localize the da Vinci instruments tips in the TRUS volume at multiple locations. After registration, the TRUS imaging plane can track the da Vinci tool tips in order to display their location relative to the internal structures seen in ultrasound. The method for direct registration of 3D TRUS to da Vinci stereo-camera system [3] was also implemented in order to overlay TRUS images to the surgeon's camera view at the correct spatial location for improved guidance.

2   Material and Methods

Experimental Setup and Clinical Setting: A 10-month-old male hound weighing 27 kg was used in this IACUC-approved study (Institutional Animal Care and Use Committee). Following a lower bowel prep, the anaesthetized animal was placed on the OR table in a 40-degree Trendelenburg position. Before docking the da Vinci surgical robot, the TRUS robot was attached to the OR table using the MicroTouch Brachytherapy stabilizer passive arm (CIVCO Medical Solutions, Kalona, IA), which was adjusted for the TRUS to provide optimal transversal and sagittal images of the animal's prostate as done in standard brachytherapy procedures (Figure 1). A Sonix TABLET ultrasound machine

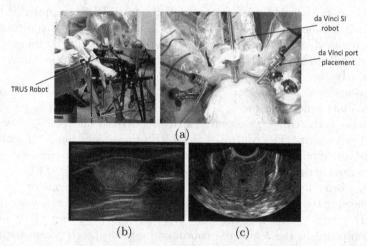

Fig. 1. The clinical setup and TRUS images of the canine's prostate: (a)TRUS robot attached to the OR table in Trendelenburg position with the da Vinci robot docked to the table and da Vinci ports are placed as in RALRP. (b)Sagittal plane TRUS image of the prostate at elevational depth of 4 cm. (c)Transverse plane TRUS image.

(Ultrasonix Medical Corp., Richmond, BC) with a bi-plane TRUS transducer was used for imaging. All TRUS volumes were captured using the 128-element 55 mm long linear BPL9-5/55 array with transmit frequency of 6.6 MHz and imaging depth of 4.0 cm. They were acquired using an 80-degree rotary sweep about the probe axis, and contained 220 images at increments of 0.36 degrees. Image capture time was 8.8 seconds per volume. The surgeons placed the da Vinci ports in the recommended pattern for RALRP, taking into consideration the smaller size of the canine model. Three arms were used for the procedure, with a Large Needle Driver, Prograsp and Maryland Bi-polar forceps in the right, left and third arm respectively. A 12 mm 0-degree stereo endoscope (3.8 mm disparity) was used throughout the procedure. TilePro was used in order for the surgeon to see the ultrasound image in the da Vinci console while performing the surgery. The surgeon continued with the RALRP procedure, with the TRUS transducer in position, until the anterior surface of the prostate was visible in the stereo camera.

3D TRUS to da Vinci Stereo-Camera Registration: Because the air-tissue boundary is the only region that can be visualized in both the camera and ultrasound image, a direct registration method as described in [3] was performed using a drop-in registration tool consisting of a machined stainless steel plate, with angled handles designed for easy grasping by the da Vinci needle driver instruments. The tool has three camera markers on one face, and three ball-bearing ball fiducials on the other face (Figure 2). The registration tool was inserted in the abdominal cavity through one of the ports, and placed on the prostate surface, where all three camera markers and the ultrasound fiducials were visible in the camera and US images, respectively. The coordinates of the three camera markers in the camera frame were detected by the stereo triangulation. The spherical fiducial corresponding to each marker was localized manually in the TRUS volumes by clicking on the appropriate B-Mode images. A homogeneous transformation between the two frames was found using least squares [3]. In order to accurately localize the markers on the registration tool, a standard camera calibration [4] was completed before capturing the camera images. The registration tool was repositioned four times in order to acquire 12 paired ultrasound fiducial and camera marker locations. In order to validate

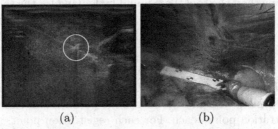

(a)   (b)

Fig. 2. (a)US image of the registration tool pressed on the anterior surface of the prostate, where the fiqucial in the US image is circled. (b)Camera image of the surgical site through the da Vinci console.

the registration method and to determine its accuracy, three pairs (representing one registration tool position) or six pairs (representing two registration tool positions) of ultrasound fiducials and camera markers were used to find the homogeneous transformation. The remaining points were used as target points to calculate the target registration error (TRE), defined as the distance between the point in camera space and the ultrasound fiducial point *transformed* into camera space. Registration accuracy results are listed in Table 1.

TRUS to da Vinci Instrument Registration: The surgeon was asked to press the tool tip of a da Vinci instrument against the prostate surface while a full TRUS volume was being acquired. The tool tip is visible as a hyperechoic focal point in the B-Mode image. To manually find the tool tip, first the angle of the TRUS imaging plane is selected. Then the tool tip axial and lateral coordinates are selected in this plane. The tip location relative to the TRUS coordinate system is obtained by transforming these cylindrical coordinates to Cartesian ones. The tool tip location relative to the robot coordinate system is also known from the Research API provided by Intuitive Surgical [6], providing three constraint equations for the homogeneous transformation relating the da Vinci coordinate system to that of the TRUS. Multiple constraints are obtained by repeating the process. $N = 12$ different target locations and corresponding volumes were acquired. For $n = 100$ iterations, $N_f = 4$ point pairs were picked at random and a least squares problem was solved to find the registration homogeneous transformation. The remaining $N_t = N - N_f = 8$ target locations were used to calculate the TRE, defined as the error between the location of the tool tips and the transformed points from the ultrasound volumes. To determine the inter-subject variation (ISV) in fiducial localization and analyze its effect on TRE, four different ultrasound users were asked to localize the tool tip in each of the $N = 12$ B-mode TRUS volumes we acquired. The TRE and Fiducial Registration Errors (FRE) in all three anatomical directions and RMS values for each user, as well as the mean over all users, are reported in Table 2.

3D TRUS to da Vinci Instrument Registration Using Automatic Tool Localization: In addition to the manual localization, the 3D automatic tool tip localization algorithm developed in [11], was also used on these $N = 12$ volumes. In this method the tool tip is found by looking for the tool tip signature on the surface (Figure 3) in the volume. The automatic detection results were compared to those obtained manually by four observers. The results can be found in Table 3.

Registration Timing: To determine the ease with which the above registrations can be performed, we asked the surgeon to perform four timed registrations using four registration points each. For each registration point, the tool tip location was found manually in the ultrasound volume. Often the surgeon would gently move the tool tip to confirm the correct tool tip location. After each registration, the automatic tracking was activated and the surgeon was asked to

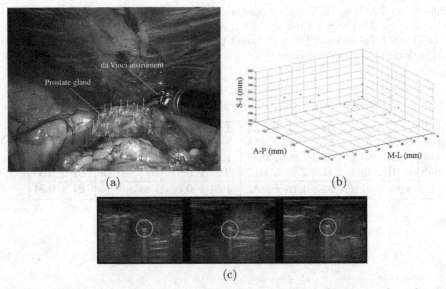

Fig. 3. (a) Camera image of the surgical site through the da Vinci console and spatial locations of the instrument tips scattered on the surface of the prostate. (b) The da Vinci intrument tip locations were spread on the surface of the prostate to achieve an accurate registration across the entire prostate gland. (c) US images of the da Vinci instrument tip pressed on the anterior prostate surface at different points.

move the tool tip to an additional 10 points on the surface of the prostate. For each location, the corresponding TRUS angle was recorded, then the tracking was temporarily deactivated and the points were located manually by adjusting the TRUS angle. The error in this measurement is shown in Table 4.

3   Results

3D TRUS to da Vinci Stereo-Camera Registration: Table 1 lists mean TRE and FRE when one or two registration tool positions are used for registering the TRUS to the camera. Since 12 point-pairs in the camera and US frames were collected and could be used for registration; the results are averaged over all combinations of 3 fiducials out of 12 points (one tool position), and all combinations of 6 out of 12 points (two tool positions).

Table 1. 3D TRUS to da Vinci stereo-camera registration accuracy

Tool positions	Number of fiducials (N_f)	Number of targets (N_t)	Mean FRE (mm)	Mean TRE (mm)
1	3	9	0.68 ± 0.42	3.91 ± 1.23
2	6	6	0.95 ± 0.38	2.73 ± 1.06

Table 2. 3D TRUS to da Vinci surgical tool registration accuracy (Manual tool tip localization in 3D TRUS). TRE and FRE are calculated for ($n = 100$) iterations, ($N_f = 4$) tool tip points and ($N_t = 8$) target points with 4 manual tool tip localization trials perfomed by 4 different users.

	$TRE_{AP}(mm)$	$TRE_{SI}(mm)$	$TRE_{ML}(mm)$	Mean TRE (mm)	Mean FRE (mm)
Subject 1	1.96 ± 1.04	1.66 ± 0.54	1.78 ± 0.85	1.86 ± 0.80	0.86 ± 0.44
Subject 2	1.93 ± 0.52	1.62 ± 0.58	1.72 ± 0.70	1.76 ± 0.61	0.97 ± 0.97
Subject 3	1.94 ± 1.09	1.67 ± 0.99	1.80 ± 0.92	1.81 ± 0.99	0.91 ± 0.35
Subject 4	2.19 ± 1.31	2.07 ± 1.17	2.07 ± 0.97	2.11 ± 1.15	1.02 ± 0.38
Average	2.01 ± 0.99	1.75 ± 0.82	1.84 ± 0.86	1.88 ± 0.88	0.94 ± 0.54

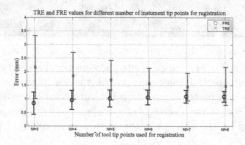

Fig. 4. TRE and FRE values for different number of tool tip points used for registration. As the number of fiducials increase, TRE decreases. We suggest using 6 fiducials in clinical applications.

TRUS to da Vinci Instrument Registration with Manual Fiducial Localization: Table 2 lists the mean values for TRE and FRE during TRUS robot to da Vinci instrument registration. A total of 12 TRUS volumes and da Vinci API point-pairs were collected. Errors are represented in the anatomical frame of the patient (Anterior-Posterior (AP), Superior-Inferior (SI), Medial-Lateral (ML)). Mean values of FRE and TRE and their standard deviations were calculated for each combination of (N_t,N_f) for 100 iterations and the results are plotted in Figure 4. As can be seen from this figure, as N_f increases, both the mean and the standard deviation of the TRE decreases. Based on this analysis, the number of fiducials suggested for this registration is $N_f = 6$.

Table 3. 3D TRUS to da Vinci surgical tool registration accuracy (Automatic tool tip localization in 3D TRUS). Mean TRE and FRE for ($n = 100$) iterations, with ($N_f = 4$) tool tip points and ($N_t = 8$) target points, FLE in (x, y) and (θ) and inter-subject variations calculated for 4 users.

FRE (mm)	TRE (mm)	$FLE_{(x,y)}$ (mm)	FLE_θ (deg)	$ISV_{(x,y)}$ (mm)	ISV_θ (deg)
1.56 ± 0.57	2.68 ± 0.98	2.91 ± 0.90	1.48 ± 0.70	3.55 ± 0.34	1.62 ± 0.39

Table 4. Automatic da Vinic tool tip tracking accuracy

	Tracking error (deg)	Mean TRE (mm)	Time
Registration Trial 1	1.47 ± 0.83	1.78 ± 0.65	120s
Registration Trial 2	1.63 ± 1.22	2.00 ± 1.04	90s
Registration Trial 3	1.95 ± 1.28	2.11 ± 1.17	111s
Registration Trial 4	1.58 ± 1.63	1.83 ± 0.76	64s
Average	1.65 ± 1.24	1.93 ± 0.90	96s

TRUS to da Vinci Instrument Registration Using Automatic Tool Localization: The TRE and FRE obtained with automatic fiducial localization technique compared to manual localization are listed in Table 3. The table includes the TRUS imaging plane angle (θ) localization error, and the localization error ((x, y)(θ)=lateral, axial) in the plane at θ. The fiducial localization error of the algorithm and the inter-subject variations (ISV) seen during manual localization are also reported.

Registration Timing: The tracking accuracy for the four timed registration trials are reported in Table 4. TRE values were also calculated for each registration. All registrations were completed in under 2 minutes with an average registration time of 96 seconds. Throughout the registration experiments and the surgery, TRUS images were streamed into the da Vinci console for real-time guidance. Figure 5 shows the TilePro and camera images inside the da Vinci console, when the automatic tool tracking is activated and the TRUS image follows the da Vinci tool tip.

4 Discussion

In this set of experiments, we tested and validated the intraoperative use of a robotic TRUS manipulator for RALRP procedures. The TRUS robot is based on a small modification to a standard brachytherapy stabilizer which is available in almost any hospital where brachytherapy is performed. Hospital staff are familiar

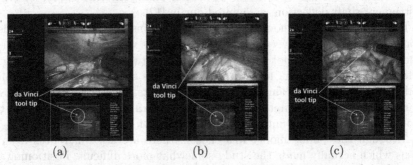

(a)   (b)   (c)

Fig. 5. TilePro images inside the surgeon console while the automatic tool tracking is activated. The da Vinci instrument tip is visible in both camera and ultrasound images.

with the set-up and positioning of the transducer on the stabilizer with respect to the patient.

Registration of the TRUS robot to the da Vinci camera showed a mean TRE of 2.73 mm when using two tool positions. This is about 1mm larger than the error reported using the system in phantoms [3]. Unlike [3], which used a cross-wire phantom to compute TRE, the current approach uses point-pairs of camera markers/ultrasound fiducials at different locations of the registration tool. This approach is more clinically practical but may lead to higher registration errors. The tight space within the pelvic cavity limited the registration tool placements that we could use. To avoid this problem, a more compact registration tool should be designed in the future.

During the TRUS to da Vinci tool registration, a TRE of 1.88 ± 0.88 mm was achieved. This is on par with the results from [3] when using a PVC prostate phantom. It is pointed out by Ukimura *et al.* [13] that the mean distance between the NVB and the lateral edge of the prostate ranged from 1.9 ± 0.8 mm at the prostate apex, to 2.5 ± 0.8 mm at the base. This is suggestive of the required accuracy of a guidance system since one major aspect of the system is to accurately localize the NVB. Currently the error in our TRUS to camera registration is slightly larger, but the error between the da Vinci tools and the TRUS is within the range reported in [13].

We believe that a large part of the error in the camera to TRUS registration was due to the difficulty of accurate camera calibration, which presently requires that the camera be taken off the robot. The da Vinci stereo camera has a disparity of 3.8 mm, meaning that the depth measurement calculated from the differences between the left and right images is very sensitive to calibration. For both registration approaches (to camera and to tool), some of the registration error may also be due to the limited localization accuracy of the fiducials within the US images. While subjects were instructed on the best way of picking the fiducial edges as described in [7], they had higher variance in localizing the fiducials than the automatic method. The use of an automated algorithm would also mean that no additional personnel would be needed in the OR in order for the tracking to be activated. For the TRUS to da Vinci tool registration error, another contributing factor is the tool tip localization error from the da Vinci API, which has been reported to be within 2mm. Another source of error is instrument shaft deflection, as pointed out in [12].

Timing results have shown that the da Vinci instrument to TRUS registration could be completed very quickly and would be valid throughout the surgery since neither the TRUS nor the da Vinci coordinate systems will be moving. We determined that using six tool tip positions gives the best TRE with minimal added benefit derived from further measurements. This would increase registration time by approximately 20 seconds. Camera to TRUS registration tools should be similar, not counting the time required for camera calibration.

Although the canine model was chosen, there are key differences from humans which actually made the study somewhat more difficult. Positioning with a human patient does not usually put extensive pressure on the distal end of the transducer, but in the canine case, there was a larger amount of force on the transducer which could cause errors in TRUS rotation during TRUS volume acquisition and also in fiducial lozalization in TRUS images.

5   Conclusions

We have presented the validation of two intraoperative registration methods that can be used during RALRP for image guidance and surgical navigation. Both methods use the air-tissue boundary as a common interface for the da Vinci robot and the ultrasound images. The da Vinci camera to TRUS registration is the first step in creating an augmented reality navigation system for da Vinci surgery (3D image overlays in the surgeon's console). Using the kinematics of the robot, we were able to register the da Vinci coordinate system with that of the TRUS robot. This was achieved quickly and efficiently with surgeons new to this concept. All registration errors were within the scope of the clinical setting and the constraints of the ultrasound imaging system. Surgeons even suggested approaches on how to distribute the registration points (2 points at the prostate base, 2 points at mid-gland and 2 points at the apex) to make the process more efficient and maintain registration accuracy across the prostate. We have demonstrated that these registration methods work effectively in an *in-vivo* environment. The camera registration tool would need to be modified specifically for a clinical environment, while the da Vinci kinematic registration is ready for clinical testing. We have submitted our application to human ethics and we plan to begin patient studies soon.

References

1. Tracking the rise of robotic surgery for prostate cancer. NCI Cancer Bulletin 8(16) (2011)
2. Adebar, T., Salcudean, S., Mahdavi, S., Moradi, M., Nguan, C., Goldenberg, L.: A robotic system for intra-operative trans-rectal ultrasound and ultrasound elastography in radical prostatectomy. In: Taylor, R.H., Yang, G.-Z. (eds.) IPCAI 2011. LNCS, vol. 6689, pp. 79–89. Springer, Heidelberg (2011)
3. Adebar, T., Yip, M., Salcudean, S., Rohling, R., Nguan, C., Goldenberg, L.: Registration of 3d ultrasound to laparoscopic stereo cameras through an air-tissue boundary. IEEE Transactions on Medical Imaging 31(11), 2133–2142 (2012)
4. Bouguet, J.Y.: Camera calibration toolbox. Available online (2010)
5. Price, D.T., Chari, R.S., Neighbors, J.D., et al.: Laparoscopic radical prostatectomy in canine model. Journal of Laparoscopic Surgery 6(6), 405–412 (1996)
6. DiMaio, S., Hasser, C.: The da vinci reseach interface, pp. 626–634 (2008)
7. Hacihaliloglu, I., Abugharbieh, R., Hodgson, A.J., Rohling, R.N.: Bone surface localization in ultrasound using image phase-based features. Ultrasound in Medicine & Biology 35(9), 1475–1487 (2009)
8. Han, M., Stoianovici, D., Kim, C., Mozer, P., Schfer, F., Badaan, S., Vigaru, B., Tseng, K., Petrisor, D., Trock, B.: Tandem-robot assisted laparoscopic radical prostatectomy to improve the neurovascular bundle visualization: a feasibility study. Journal of Urology 77(2), 502–506 (2011)

9. Hung, A., Abreu, A., Shoji, S., Goh, A., Berger, A., Desai, M., Aron, M., Gill, I., Ukimura, O.: Robotic transrectal ultrasonography during robot-assisted radical prostatectomy. European Urology 62(2), 341–348 (2012)
10. Long, J.A., Haber, G.P., Lee, B.H., Guillotreau, J., Autorino, R., Laydner, H., Yakoubi, R., Rizkala, E., Stein, R.J., Kaouk, J.H.: Real-time robotic transrectal ultrasound navigation during robotic radical prostatectomy: initial clinical experience. Journal of Urology 80(3), 608–613 (2012)
11. Mohareri, O., Ramezani, M., Adebar, T., Abolmaesumi, P., Salcudean, S.: Automatic detection and localization of da vinci tool tips in 3D ultrasound. In: Abolmaesumi, P., Joskowicz, L., Navab, N., Jannin, P. (eds.) IPCAI 2012. LNCS, vol. 7330, pp. 22–32. Springer, Heidelberg (2012)
12. Tavakoli, M., Howe, R.D.: Haptic effects of surgical teleoperator flexibility. International Journal of Robotics Research 28(10), 1289–1302 (2009)
13. Ukimura, O., Kaouk, J., Kawauchi, A., Miki, T., Gill, I., Desai, M., Steinberg, A., Kilciler, M., Ng, C., Abreu, S., Spaliviero, M., Ramani, A.: Real-time transrectal ultrasonography during laparoscopic radical prostatectomy. Journal of Urology 172(1), 112–118 (2004)

Augmentation of Paramedian 3D Ultrasound Images of the Spine

Abtin Rasoulian[1], Robert N. Rohling[1,2], and Purang Abolmaesumi[1]

[1] Department of Electrical and Computer Engineering
[2] Department of Mechanical Engineering,
University of British Columbia, Vancouver, B.C., Canada
{abtinr,rohling,purang}@ece.ubc.ca

Abstract. The blind placement of an epidural needle is among the most difficult regional anesthetic techniques. The challenge is to insert the needle in the mid-sagittal plane and to avoid overshooting the needle into the spinal cord. Prepuncture 2D ultrasound scanning has been introduced as a reliable tool to localize the target and facilitate epidural needle placement. Ideally, real-time ultrasound should be used *during* needle insertion. However, several issues inhibit the use of standard 2D ultrasound, including the obstruction of the puncture site by the ultrasound probe, low visibility of the target in ultrasound images, and increased pain due to longer needle trajectory. An alternative is to use 3D ultrasound imaging, where the needle and target could be visible within the same reslice of a 3D volume; however, novice ultrasound users (i.e., many anesthesiologists) still have difficulty interpreting ultrasound images of the spine and identifying the target epidural space. In this paper, we propose to augment 3D ultrasound images by registering a multi-vertebrae statistical shape+pose model. We use such augmentation for enhanced interpretation of the ultrasound and identification of the mid-sagittal plane for the needle insertion. Validation is performed on synthetic data derived from the CT images, and 64 *in vivo* ultrasound volumes.

Keywords: multi-vertebrae shape+pose model, 3D ultrasound, Gaussian mixture model-based registration.

1 Introduction

Epidurals are a form of regional anesthesia commonly used in obstetrics during labour and delivery, and they are effective alternatives to general anesthesia for cesarean delivery. Epidurals involve the insertion of a needle between the vertebrae into a space called the epidural space (see Fig. 1a). The use of epidurals has increased over the past few decades but conventional epidural techniques continue to have a failure rate in the range of 6-20% [4], meaning the patient has inadequate or no pain relief.

Before the procedure, no detailed knowledge about the individual patient's spinal anatomy is available to guide the anesthesiologist. Therefor, epidurals are traditionally guided by palpation of surface landmarks to identify an appropriate intervertebral space and to select a skin puncture site along the midline of

D. Barratt et al. (Eds.): IPCAI 2013, LNCS 7915, pp. 51–60, 2013.
© Springer-Verlag Berlin Heidelberg 2013

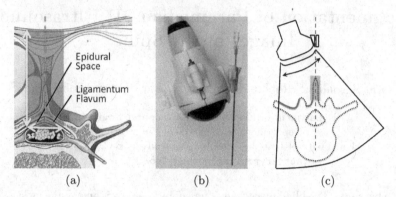

(a)   (b)   (c)

Fig. 1. a) Midline sagittal insertion of the needle. The horizontal arrow shows the epidural width and the vertical arrow shows the epidural depth. b) 3D motorized ultrasound probe equipped with a needle guide. c) The relative positions of the 3D ultrasound probe, needle and vertebra in superior-inferior view. The arrow shows the sweep direction. The probe should be placed to align the needle path (dashed blue line) with the mid-sagittal plane. The red line shows the visible part of the vertebrae in ultrasound images. No echoes appear on the gray area since the spinous process surface is not orthogonal to the transducer.

the spine. The loss-of-resistance technique is normally used to confirm that the needle tip has reached the epidural space. This technique involves attaching a saline-filled syringe to the needle and applying pressure during needle insertion and then feeling the loss-of-resistance to saline injection when the needle tip enters the epidural space. The most common complication (0.5% to 2.5% [16]) arises from overshoot and accidental puncture of the dura mater surrounding the spinal cord and leakage of cerebral spinal fluid, which leads to side effects for patients, such as post dural puncture headache.

To reduce complications, ultrasound imaging has been proposed since it poses no known risk to the patient, making it the only modality that is feasible for obstetric anesthesiology. 2D ultrasound imaging has been demonstrated as a pre-puncture tool for measuring the distance from the skin to the epidural space (referred to as the epidural depth) and to help decide the puncture site [8].

Ideally, ultrasound would also be used *during* needle insertion to visually confirm the needle progressing toward and then entering the epidural space correctly. Unfortunately, real-time guidance of a midline needle insertion is hindered by the fact that a standard 2D ultrasound transducer obscures the puncture site, and moving the transducer to the side makes it impossible to view both the needle tip and the target together. The usual image-guidance solutions based on tracking of both the needle and the ultrasound transducer do not work in this application. The tracking sensor would need to be either mounted on the base of the needle, which reduces the accuracy due to needle bending, or placed inside the needle close to its tip, which prohibits the standard procedure of loss-of-resistance since the sensor does not allow passage of the saline.

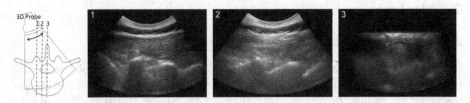

Fig. 2. Three parallel slices extracted from the 3D ultrasound image. Arrow shows the sweep direction. Planes are spaced 10 mm from each other. Ideally, the anesthesiologist should perform the needle injection in the third plane which does not include strong features. The first plane shows the facet joints whereas the second plane shows the laminae. The planes are also hard for novice users to distinguish the anatomy in the ultrasound, making needle guidance difficult.

A solution to these problems has been developed using a 3D motorized ultrasound transducer equipped with a needle guide (see Figure 1b and 1c) [13]. 3D ultrasound is widely used in obstetrics and has several advantages such as easier diagnosis of cleft palate [17]. 3D ultrasound also has the potential to improve epidural catheterization and operation orientation of the vertebral column [1]. In our solution, a virtual anterior-posterior plane (hereafter referred to as a reslice plane) containing the needle path is extracted from volumes captured in real time by the transducer. Placing the transducer in a paramedian plane and consequently placing the needle in midline, the reslice plane depicts both the needle and the epidural space. Initial experiments on animals have shown the feasibility of this approach [13], but there are still limitations of this technique. First, the ultrasound images are hard to interpret and require extensive training. Second, detection of the mid-sagittal plane is not trivial due to a lack of significant image features in this plane (see Fig. 2).

In the absence of pre-operative CT image for the majority of obstetric cases, augmentation of 3D ultrasound has been explored previously by registering a statistical shape model of a single vertebra [15]. In that study, the ultrasound volumes were acquired with the probe centered on the midline and bony features from both side of the vertebrae were visible. In this paper we modify that approach and make two main contributions. First, we demonstrate construction of the multi-vertebrae shape+pose statistical model and its registration to ultrasound volumes of the spine. Second, we perform the registration to single-sided paramedian ultrasound volumes. Registration is challenging due to the lack of echoes on the contra-lateral side, and thus a lack of information on the symmetric shape of the vertebrae.

In summary, the model is registered to the ultrasound images based on echoes that are typically visible in such ultrasound images, i.e. laminae, articular processes, and transverse processes of one side of the vertebrae. We use the registered model to interpret the echoes in the ultrasound images and to predict the mid-sagittal plane. We validate our registration technique on synthetic data and 64 *in vivo* ultrasound volumes.

2   Methods

2.1   Construction of the Multi-vertebrae Model

Several techniques have been proposed for construction of multi-object statistical models [2,9,5,10,12]. In some of these techniques, the pose statistics are neglected by implicitly representing them in the shape statistics. This representation leads to two major issues: first, the pose statistics are not necessarily correlated with the shape statistics, since they depend on external factors such as the position and orientation of the patient during data acquisition. Second, the shape deformations are assumed to lie on a Euclidean space. On the other hand, the poses are represented by similarity transformations, i.e. rigid+scale transformations. These transformations form a Lie group, which is a Riemannian manifold where analysis performed in Euclidean space is not applicable [6]. To address this problem, we adapt a technique proposed by Bossa and Olmos [2] to generate a statistical multi-vertebrae shape+pose model.

A Lie group G is a group and a differentiable manifold where multiplication and inversion are smooth. The tangent space at the identity element is called Lie algebra, $\mathfrak{g}$. The exponential mapping, $\mathfrak{g} : \exp(x) \to G$, and its inverse, logarithm mapping $G : \log(x) \to \mathfrak{g}$, are used to map elements in the tangent space into G and vice versa.

Analogous to principal components in the Euclidean space, Principal Geodesics (PG), are defined for Lie groups. The approximation as suggested By Fletcher *et al.* [6] is as follows: for a set of elements, $x_1, \ldots, x_n$, the mean, μ, is found using an iterative approach. Principal Component Analysis (PCA) is then applied to the residuals in the Lie algebra, $\log(\mu^{-1}x_i)$. The results are orthonormal principal components, v_l, which give the PGs by exponential mapping, $\mu \exp(v_l)$.

Assume that the training set contains N instances of an ensemble of L anatomies (in this case L vertebrae), each represented by a point set as its boundary. Initially, a group-wise Gaussian mixture model (GMM)-based registration technique [14] is used to establish dense correspondences across the training set. Generalized Procrustes analysis is then used to generate the mean shape for all the anatomies, and their transformation, $\mathbf{T}_{n,l}$, to each instance. The transformation, $\mathbf{T}_{n,l}$, is the similarity transformation from the lth anatomy of the mean shape to the corresponding anatomy of the nth instance. The transformation for all anatomies are concatenated and PGs are then extracted. The results are principal geodesics, which can separately be written for each anatomy: $\mu_l^p \exp(\mathbf{v}_{k,l}^p)$. Shapes also form a Lie group [2] and similarly shapes' PGs can be represented by $\mu_l^s \exp(\mathbf{v}_{k,l}^s)$. Note that we use superscript "s" and "p" to differentiate between shape and pose related variables, respectively.

2.2   Enhancement of the Ultrasound Images

A preprocessing step is performed on the ultrasound images to extract the bone surface probability using high intensity and shadow information. To extract the

bone surface probability, we use an adaptation of a technique proposed by Foroughi *et al.* [7]. Initially, the image is filtered by Laplace of Gaussian (LoG)
kernel to extract the high intensity pixels which typically have larger probability to be on the bone surface. The result is added to the blurred image. Next,
the blurred image is convoluted by a profile highlighting the shadow beneath a
pixel. The shadow image is combined with the blurred image to generate the
bone probability map.

2.3   Registration of the Model to the Ultrasound Images

The multi-object statistical model can be instantiated by applying different
weights to the PGs and combining them. Assuming that w_k^s is the weight applied
to the kth shape PG and w_k^p is applied to the kth pose PG, the lth object of the
model can be instantiated as follows:

$$s_l = \Phi(\mathbf{w}^s, \mathbf{w}^p) = \Phi_l^p\big(\Phi_l^s(\mathbf{w}^s); \mathbf{w}^p\big), \tag{1}$$

where $\Phi_l^p(.; \mathbf{w}^p)$ and $\Phi_l^s(.)$ denote a similarity transformation and a shape, respectively, which are built by a combination of the pose and shape PGs with
corresponding weights:

$$\Phi^p(.; \mathbf{w}^p) = \mu_l^p \prod_{k=1}^{K} \exp(w_k^p \mathbf{v}_{k,l}^p) \quad \text{and} \quad \Phi_l^s(\mathbf{w}^s) = \exp_{\mu_l^s}(\sum_{k=1}^{K} w_k^s \mathbf{v}_{k,l}^s). \tag{2}$$

The registration is performed using a GMM-based technique proposed earlier [14].
In this iterative technique, soft-correspondences are established between surface
of the model and the target that is represented by a point set. Assume that
the *correspondance* function, $P(\mathbf{x}_n^l, \mathbf{y}_m)$, is defined for the nth point of the lth
anatomy on the model, $\mathbf{x}_n^l$, and the mth point of the target, $\mathbf{y}_m$, and has a value
between 0 and 1. The point set $\mathbf{Y}$ constitutes a partial surface of the vertebrae
and is extracted from the ultrasound images as explained in the previous section.
Additionally, the bone surface probability extracted from the ultrasound images
is already integrated into the correspondence function.

The model is then instantiated and rigidly transformed to minimize the
following objective function:

$$Q = \sum_{l=1}^{L} \sum_{m,n=1}^{M,N} P(\mathbf{x}_n^l|\mathbf{y}_m)\|\mathbf{y}_m - (\mathbf{R}\Phi(\mathbf{x}_n^l; \mathbf{w}^s, \mathbf{w}^p) + \mathbf{t})\|^2 + \gamma^s\mathbf{\Gamma^s}\mathbf{w}^s + \gamma^p\mathbf{\Gamma^p}\mathbf{w}^p, \tag{3}$$

where the two latter terms are the regularization over the PGs weights, and
matrices $\mathbf{\Gamma^s}$ and $\mathbf{\Gamma^p}$ are diagonal with elements $1/\lambda^s$ and $1/\lambda^p$, the corresponding
eigenvalues of the shape and the pose PGs, respectively. The matrices $\mathbf{R}$ and
$\mathbf{t}$ are the rotation and translation of the rigid transformation, respectively. The
optimization is performed using the Quasi-Newton method.

Note that the objective function is minimized with respect to the points of the model that are visible in ultrasound volumes, i.e. laminae, articular processes and transverse processes of one side only (see Fig. 1b).

This is the key challenge. Once registered, the model is used later to estimate the location of the mid-sagittal plane. This is performed by fitting a plane to the tip of the spinous processes and most anterior point of the vertebral body.

3   Experiments and Results

3.1   Multi-vertebrae Shape+Pose Model

Training data for construction of the multi-vertebrae model consisted of lumbar (L1-L5) vertebrae of 32 patients, some with mild scolisis. Written informed consent was obtained from all patients. Manual CT segmentations were performed semi-automatically using ITK-SNAP. For each subject, three independent segmentations (performed by three different users) were averaged using majority voting to form the final segmentation, then triangulated using the marching cubes algorithm.

The statistical shape+pose model was reconstructed using the technique presented in the previous section. The first 10 modes capture 97% of pose variations and 70% of shape variations. The model is capable of reconstructing an unseen observation with distance error below 1.5 mm by using the first 10 modes of the variation.

3.2   Synthetic Data

To assess the performance of the registration of one side of the model to the corresponding ultrasound images in an ideal scenario, we constructed a synthetic data set using 32 CT scans and performed leave-one-out experiments. For each CT scan, the model is constructed using all other CT images and is registered to a surface extracted from one side of L1-L4 vertebrae of the target, including the laminae, articular processes and transverse processes. The surface error is then computed for the entire vertebrae and results in an RMS distance error of 2.2±0.6 mm. Fig. 3 shows the distance error overlaid on the model. As expected, the registration error is smallest near the anatomy involved in the registration and increases further away. The registration error is largest around the spinous process since its shape is not correlated with laminae and transverse processes. This error is however not critical since the epidural space is not close to the spinous process and does not affect needle insertion. Interestingly, the error is equally distributed in the other regions, i.e. laminae and articular processes on the opposite side and vertebral body.

The registered model is then used to estimate the mid-sagittal plane and is compared against the mid-sagittal plane extracted from manual segmentation. The normals of the two planes differ by 4.4±2.6 degrees, and the location of the epidural space in the registered model differs from the mid-sagittal plane of

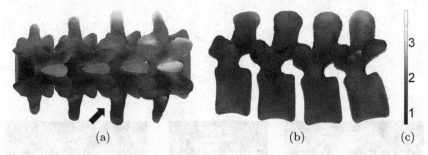

Fig. 3. Distance error overlaid on the model in the a) anterior-posterior and b) left-to-right view. The arrow points to the side used in the registration.

Table 1. The registration error of the model to the paramedian volume. Values are given as mean±std (mm).

		L1-L2	L2-L3	L3-L4	L4-L5	All
Registration side	RMS	2.0±0.3	3.0±1.7	2.5±0.9	3.0±1.1	2.6±1.2
	Haussdorf	3.7±1.0	6.8±4.3	4.6±2.7	5.1±2.8	5.0±3.1
Contra-lateral side	RMS	4.4±2.0	4.0±2.0	3.9±1.4	3.5±1.1	3.9±1.7
	Haussdorf	7.1±3.2	7.4±3.0	6.7±2.7	6.1±3.0	6.8±3.0

the manual segmentation by 1.3±1.2 mm. As we will mention in the Discussion, these errors effectively convey the ability to register the model using only a few features on only one side of the vertebral anatomy.

3.3 *In Vivo* Data

3D ultrasound volumes were captured by an expert sonographer using a Sonix Touch ultrasound machine (Ultrasonix, Medical Corp, Richmond, BC) with a curvilinear 3D transducer, operating at 3.3 MHz with depth of 7.0 cm. 80 frames were captured for each volume to have a 60 degree field of view. The 3D probe was tracked using an EM tracker (pciBird, Ascension Technology Corp., Burlington, VT, USA) and was calibrated using double N-wire phantom with an RMS error of 1.7 mm [3]. The purpose of tracking is only for validation of the model registration to the volumes on the contra-lateral side and for measurement of the true mid-sagittal plane.

Written consent was obtained from eight volunteers. Ultrasound volumes were acquired in the prone position. For each subject, the intervertebral levels were found using 2D ultrasound and were marked on the skin. A magnetic sensor (referred to as the reference) was attached on the skin above the T12 vertebra to track the patient's movement. We assumed that the spine curvature does not change during the entire scan. Four intervertebral levels (L1-L2, L2-L3, L3-L4, and L4-5) were scanned. Three volumes were acquired from each level (see Fig. 4), one paramedian volume from each side and one centered on the mid-sagittal plane (referred to as the *centered volume*). Note that bony features are

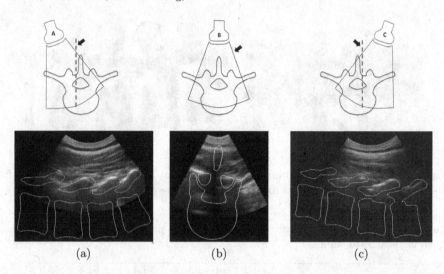

(a)   (b)   (c)

Fig. 4. Three volumes are acquired from each intervertebral level. Arrows show the plane visualized in each case. a) The model is registered to this paramedian volume (volume A). The red dashed line shows the sagittal slice of this volume shown together with the registered model. b) A transverse view of the centered volume (volume B) augmented with the registered model. c) A sagittal view of the contra-lateral volume (volume C) augmented with the registered model.

Table 2. Error between the two mid-sagittal planes, one estimated from the registered model, and one extracted from the centered 3D US volume. Distance is defined as the distance between two planes at the epidural depth.

	L1-L2	L2-L3	L3-L4	L4-L5	All
Normal (degree)	6.4±2.4	13.0±7.5	10.0±8.0	14.2±8.6	10.8±7.5
Distance (mm)	4.0±2.9	5.6±4.6	4.5±3.1	6.1±4.9	5.0±3.9

most visible in the paramedian volumes whereas the mid-sagittal plane is best detected in the centered volume. The ultrasound volumes were then transformed to the reference coordinate system using the position tracker measurements and calibration of the 3D ultrasound probe.

Registration Accuracy. The bone surfaces were manually extracted for each paramedian volume. The model was registered to one of the paramedian ultrasound volumes (e.g. volume A in Fig. 4). Examples of the registrations are shown in Fig. 5. The RMS and maximum (referred to as Haussdorf) distance between the manual segmentation of the ultrasound volume and the registered model are calculated and reported. We also reported the error between the same registered model and the paramedian ultrasound volumes acquired from the contra-lateral side (e.g. volume C in Fig. 4). Fig. 4a and 4c show an example of the registration. Results are given in Table 1. As expected the error is larger on the contra-lateral side, but remains below 4.4 mm.

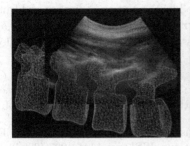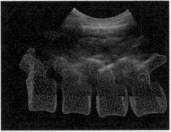

Fig. 5. Examples of the registration. The multi-vertebrae model is capable of capturing different sizes, shapes and poses of vertebrae.

Detection of the Mid-Sagittal Plane. The mid-sagittal plane is detected by fitting a plane to the points acquired by marking the symmetric features of vertebral anatomy (i.e. laminae and transverse processes) and taking their average. The manually extracted plane is compared against the mid-sagittal plane extracted from the registered model. Similar to synthetic data, the angle between these two planes and their separation at the depth of the epidural space is reported. Results are given in Table 2. Fig. 4b shows an example of the registered model together with the centered volume.

4   Discussion and Conclusion

It is expected that the multi-vertebrae model will be used to augment the ultrasound image interpretation and to predict the mid-sagittal plane of the spine, but not replace the standard technique for epidural needle placement such as loss-of-resistance. In this pilot study, we have demonstrated that the errors for registering the model to single-sided ultrasound volumes of the human spine have an average of 2.6 mm on the registration side and 3.9 mm on average on the contra-lateral side.

The width of the ligamentum flavum covering the epidural space is reported to be 6.8 ± 1.9 [11]. The epidural depth varies between patients, and increases with obesity. In our experiments, the maximum epidural depth was 47 mm. Given these numbers and referring to Fig. 1a, the safe needle insertion zone (represented by the gray area) confine the proper needle insertion to an angle of less than 8 degrees and 6.8 mm distance to the mid-sagittal plane. This suggests that the proposed method for mid-sagittal plane estimation has the potential for successful midline epidural injection. The results can be further improved by better edge enhancement in the ultrasound images and also using larger training set used for the construction of the model.

The current unoptimized MATLAB code requires 53 seconds to register the multi-vertebrae shape+pose model to 3D ultrasound images. Since the ultimate goal of this work is to visualize the ultrasound reslice augmented with the model in real-time, our future work involve optimizing the code in C++ to achieve clinically acceptable speeds.

Acknowledgments. This work is funded by the Natural Sciences and Engineering Research Council and Canadian Institutes for Health Research. The authors would also like to thank Victoria A. Lessoway for helping with data collection.

References

1. Belavy, D., Ruitenberg, M., Brijball, R.: Feasibility study of real-time three-/four-dimensional ultrasound for epidural catheter insertion. British Journal of Anaesthesia 107(3), 438–445 (2011)
2. Bossa, M., Olmos, S.: Multi-object statistical pose+shape models. In: IEEE International Symposium on Biomedical Imaging, ISBI, pp. 1204–1207 (2007)
3. Chen, T.K., Thurston, A.D., Ellis, R.E., Abolmaesumi, P.: A real-time freehand ultrasound calibration system with automatic accuracy feedback and control. Ultrasound in Medicine & Biology 35(1), 79–93 (2009)
4. Coq, G.L., Ducot, B., Benhamou, D.: Risk factors of inadequate pain relief during epidural analgesia for labour and deliver. Anaesthesia 45, 719–723 (1998)
5. Duta, N., Sonka, M.: Segmentation and interpretation of MR brain images. an improved active shape model. IEEE TMI 17(6), 1049–1062 (1998)
6. Fletcher, P., Lu, C., Joshi, S.: Statistics of shape via principal geodesic analysis on lie groups. In: IEEE CVPR, vol. 1, pp. 95–101 (2003)
7. Foroughi, P., Boctor, E., Swartz, M., et al.: 2-D ultrasound bone segmentation using dynamic programming. In: IEEE Ultras Symp., pp. 2523–2526 (2007)
8. Grau, T., Bartusseck, E., Conradi, R., et al.: Ultrasound imaging improves learning curves in obstetric epidural anesthesia: a preliminary study. Canadian Journal of Anesthesia 50(10), 1047–1050 (2003)
9. Khallaghi, S., et al.: Registration of a statistical shape model of the lumbar spine to 3D ultrasound images. In: Jiang, T., Navab, N., Pluim, J.P.W., Viergever, M.A. (eds.) MICCAI 2010, Part II. LNCS, vol. 6362, pp. 68–75. Springer, Heidelberg (2010)
10. Lu, C., Pizer, S.M., Joshi, S., Jeong, J.: Statistical multi-object shape models. International Journal of Computer Vision 75(3), 387–404 (2007)
11. Nickalls, R., Kokri, M.: The width of the posterior epidural space in obstetric patients. Anaesthesia 41(4), 432–433 (1986)
12. Okada, T., Yokota, K., Hori, M., Nakamoto, M., Nakamura, H., Sato, Y.: Construction of hierarchical multi-organ statistical atlases and their application to multi-organ segmentation from CT images. In: Metaxas, D., Axel, L., Fichtinger, G., Székely, G. (eds.) MICCAI 2008, Part I. LNCS, vol. 5241, pp. 502–509. Springer, Heidelberg (2008)
13. Rasoulian, A., Abolmaesumi, P., Rohling, R., Kamani, A., Charles, L., Lessoway, V.: Porcine thoracic epidural depth measurement using 3D ultrasound resliced images. In: Canadian Anesthesiologists Society Annual Meeting (2011)
14. Rasoulian, A., Rohling, R., Abolmaesumi, P.: Group-wise registration of point sets for statistical shape models. IEEE TMI 31(11), 2025–2034 (2012)
15. Rasoulian, A., Rohling, R., Abolmaesumi, P.: Probabilistic registration of an unbiased statistical shape model to ultrasound images of the spine. In: SPIE Medical Imaging, vol. 8316, pp. 83161P–1 (2012)
16. Sprigge, J., Harper, S.: Accidental dural puncture and post dural puncture headache in obstetric anaesthesia: presentation and management: A 23-year survey in a district general hospital. Anaesthesia 63(1), 36–43 (2007)
17. Steiner, H., Staudach, A., Spitzer, D., Schaffer, H.: Diagnostic techniques: Three-dimensional ultrasound in obstetrics and gynaecology: technique, possibilities and limitations. Human Reproduction 9(9), 1773–1778 (1994)

3D Segmentation of Curved Needles Using Doppler Ultrasound and Vibration

Troy K. Adebar and Allison M. Okamura

Stanford University, Stanford, CA

Abstract. A method for segmenting the 3D shape of curved needles in solid tissue is described. An actuator attached to the needle outside the tissue vibrates at frequencies between 600 Hz and 6500 Hz, while 3D power Doppler ultrasound imaging is applied to detect the resulting motion of the needle shaft and surrounding tissue. The cross section of the vibrating needle is detected across the series of 2D images produced by a mechanical 3D ultrasound transducer, and the needle shape is reconstructed by fitting a 3D curve to the resulting points. The sensitivity of segmentation accuracy to tissue composition, vibration frequency, and Doppler pulse repetition frequency (PRF) was examined. Comparison with manual segmentation demonstrates that this method results in an average error of 1.09 mm in *ex vivo* tissue. This segmentation method may be useful in the future for providing feedback on curved needle shape for control of robotic needle steering systems.

Keywords: Robotic system and software, ultrasound, segmentation.

1 Introduction

Percutaneous interventions using needles allow clinicians to access anatomical targets, even those deep inside the body, with minimal trauma to the patient. This hyper-minimally invasive approach is applied to biopsy, drug delivery, brachytherapy, ablation, and many other procedures. While such percutaneous procedures are common, in some cases interference from sensitive structures or obstacles can prevent straight needles from reaching the desired target. For example, in prostate brachytherapy, pubic arch interference can restrict the placement of seeds in certain patients.

Several research groups have described methods for needle steering, in which needles are inserted through tissue along controlled curved paths (see a review in [21]). In our preferred implementation, this is achieved using a robotic system to manipulate a highly flexible needle with an asymmetric bevel tip or pre-bent distal section. As such a needle is inserted into tissue, the lateral force acting on its tip causes the needle to follow a curved path. Through a combination of needle insertion and tip rotation, the needle can be steered along a variety of paths in three-dimensional (3D) space. Path planning and image-guided control for such a needle can be performed with a robotic needle steering system.

D. Barratt et al. (Eds.): IPCAI 2013, LNCS 7915, pp. 61–70, 2013.

In current practice, needle insertions are often performed using ultrasound, CT, MR, or fluoroscopic imaging for guidance. Like human clinicians, robotic needle insertion systems require medical image feedback to achieve a satisfactory level of repeatability and accuracy. However, integration of real-time medical imaging in robotic needle steering represents a significant engineering challenge. Previous approaches have thus far avoided this by using systems that restrict the steered needle to a mostly two-dimensional (2D) path, and testing in translucent artificial tissues that allow the needle's silhouette to be imaged with optical cameras. While this approach has been useful in the development of controllers, path planning algorithms and models, methods for real-time image guidance and steering in 3D are required before needle steering can progress to *in vivo* testing and patient trials.

Because of its low cost, wide-spread availability, and real-time imaging rate, we have elected to focus on ultrasound imaging. Intraoperative ultrasound can potentially be used to provide feedback to a robotic needle steering system in several ways. First, it can be used to track the needle tip relative to an anatomical target, in order to control the needle exactly to a desired final position. Second, ultrasound can be used to monitor the curved shape of the needle shaft during insertion. This could be used, for example, to detect undesired buckling of the needle, or gather information about the interaction of the needle with tissue in order to update the mechanical models used in planning and control. In this paper we focus on segmenting the curved shape of a steerable needle from 3D ultrasound data.

1.1   Prior Work

A number of previous studies have described methods for segmenting needles from B-mode ultrasound data. Many of these methods have used some variant of the Hough or Radon transform to segment straight needles [6,7,8,17,19,27]. Other methods for straight needle segmentation include the parallel integral projection transform [4], graph cuts [3], and difference images [25]. Similar methods have also been described for segmenting curved needles. The Hough and Radon transforms, for example, can be adapted to include a parametrization of needle bending [16,18]. A projection-based algorithm for segmenting curved needles has also been proposed [1], as well as a model-based approach using RANSAC [23]. Most of the previously described methods are computationally intensive, likely requiring specialized computing hardware for real-time performance. These methods have primarily applied B-mode ultrasound, which is known to produce images with poor needle visibility, particularly when imaging at an angle [5]. Many of the methods for segmenting curved needles are appropriate for only slight curvature, whereas robotically steered needles can follow paths with radius of curvature as low as 3.4 cm in tissue [14]. Also, duty-cycle control schemes for needle steering [26] can result in paths with sections of arbitrary length having variable radii of curvature, which would make parametrization for a Hough or Radon transform difficult.

As an alternative to segmentation using B-mode data alone, we propose to apply external vibration to the needle, and use ultrasound Doppler imaging to localize the vibration. Vibrating solid objects have previously been shown to produce recognizable Doppler signals [13]. This concept has been applied to localize straight needles [2,9,12] and needle tips [11] in 2D ultrasound, as well as interventional instruments for cardiac interventions [10,20] and other applications [15,22]. (To our knowledge, this concept has not previously been applied to segment curved needles in 3DUS.) This approach is particularly well suited to robotic needle steering since the needle is already held by a robotic system, and actuators that vibrate the needle can be integrated easily.

In the study described in this paper, we used piezoelectric actuators to vibrate a steerable needle at frequencies between 600 Hz and 6500 Hz, and applied 3D power Doppler ultrasound to image the resulting motion. We applied this method to reconstruct the shape of curved needles in artificial and *ex vivo* tissues, and validated the method by comparison with manual segmentation. We examined the influence of tissue simulant, vibration frequency, and Doppler PRF. To our knowledge, this work is the first to use external vibration and 3D Doppler imaging to reconstruct the complete shape of a curved needle in tissue.

2 Methods

2.1 Segmentation Concept

Figure 1 shows a conceptual overview of our segmentation method. We assume that the general needle orientation is known. A mechanical 3D ultrasound transducer is oriented so that the needle is roughly orthogonal to the image plane as it sweeps. A piezoelectric actuator (buzzer) is used to vibrate the needle, and the resulting motion of needle and surrounding tissue produces a Doppler signal.

We segment the needle by processing the series of 2D power Doppler images generated by the 3D transducer. Two preprocessing operations are performed to remove Doppler noise: pixels with less than 10% of the maximum Doppler value are removed, and patches with less than 200 pixels of connected area are removed. (For comparison, the Doppler box was typically 160 by 130 pixels). These threshold values were determined based on comparison with manual segmentation during initial testing. After preprocessing, the image coordinates of the needle cross section are estimated based on the remaining Doppler response. We have found that the Doppler response tends to be centered on the needle cross section in the transverse direction. The transverse image coordinate of the needle is thus estimated as the centroid of the Doppler response in the transverse direction. In the axial direction, the Doppler response tends to be centered somewhat below the needle as a result of a color comet tail artifact. The axial image coordinate of the needle is thus estimated as the point that separates one quarter of the sum of the Doppler response above, and three quarters below. To define the 3D needle shape, third-order polynomial curves are fit through the cross section points to define the axial and lateral coordinates as functions of the elevational coordinate.

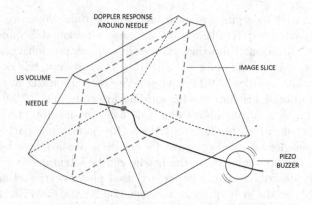

Fig. 1. Needle segmentation concept: A piezoelectric actuator attached to the needle generates vibration, resulting in a Doppler response around the needle cross section in a 2DUS image. The needle is segmented by localizing the Doppler response across the sweep of a mechanical 3DUS transducer, and fitting a curve through the resulting points.

2.2   Apparatus

Figure 2 shows our experimental apparatus.

Ultrasound Imaging. A SonixMDP ultrasound console (Ultrasonix Medical Corp., Richmond, Canada) with a convex mechanical 3D transducer (4DC7-3/40) was used for imaging. Custom software based on the Ultrasonix SDK package was used to control imaging parameters and capture images. Power Doppler imaging mode was selected over color Doppler imaging because of the lack of aliasing and reduced sensitivity to imaging angle. Pulse repetition frequency (PRF) was varied as described below in Section 2.3. The wall motion filter (WF) was set to maximum in order to minimize Doppler artifacts resulting from the motion of the imaging plane. Each sweep consisted of 61 scan-converted 2D images, captured at angular increments of approximately 0.7 degrees.

Needles. Solid stainless steel wires 0.635 mm (0.025 inches) in diameter were used as needles, with beveled tips and prebent distal sections approximately 5 mm long angled 20 degrees off axis. Piezoelectric diaphragms with four different resonant frequencies (600 Hz, CEB-20D64; 2.6 kHz, CEB-27D44; 4.6 kHz, CEB-35D26; 6.5 kHz, CEB-44D06; CUI Inc., Tualatin, OR) were soldered to the needles, and driven at their resonant frequencies by 20 V square waves created using a power supply, signal generator and simple MOSFET switching circuit. The needles were inserted into either artificial or *ex vivo* tissue, and held by a needle steering robot.

2.3   Validation Procedure

We validated our method by comparison with manual segmentation of the needle from B-mode data. To create this reference data, the center of the needle was

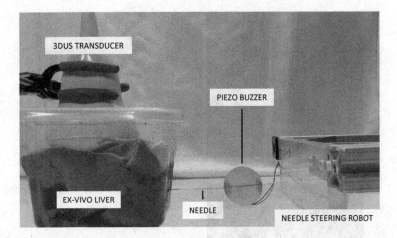

Fig. 2. Overview of experimental setup showing the 3D ultrasound transducer, an *ex vivo* bovine liver tissue sample, the piezo buzzer attached to the needle, and the needle steering robot

manually selected in all 2D B-mode images where it was visible. (The needle cross section could generally only be identified when the imaging plane was close to orthogonal to the needle, approximately 25% to 50% of the images from most sweeps.) To determine segmentation error, we measured the distance between each manually-segmented point and the reconstructed 3D needle curve within an axial-transverse plane. In order to estimate the precision of the manual segmentation, it was repeated for several test volumes, and the variation between trials was measured.

We tested the sensitivity of segmentation error to three tissue simulants, four vibration frequencies, and five Doppler PRF settings. First, the twelve possible combinations of tissue simulant and vibration frequency were tested, with needles inserted and scanned along three random curved paths for each combination. The tissue simulants were two cylindrical polyvinyl chloride (PVC) rubber phantoms and an sample of bovine liver tissue, obtained fresh from a local butcher. The formulations of the PVC were 4:1 and 1:1 Plastisol to softener, resulting in approximate elastic moduli of 33 kPa and 8.6 kPa [24]. Glass microbeads were added at a ratio of 0.025 percent by mass to create speckle. Four vibration frequencies were tested: 600 Hz, 2600 Hz, 4600 Hz, and 6500 Hz. A single PRF of 1666 Hz was used for this round of testing, with WF set to the maximum 800 Hz.

The effect of PRF was measured in a separate test using a single tissue simulant (PVC rubber with $E = 8.6$ kPa) and a single vibration frequency (2600 Hz). Five PRF settings were tested: 1428 Hz, 1666 Hz, 2000 Hz, 3333 Hz, and 6666 Hz. WF was set to maximum in each case. Again, three scans were performed for each PRF setting, with the needle inserted along a random curved path for each.

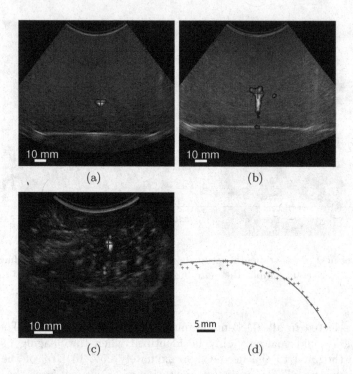

Fig. 3. Processed ultrasound images of vibrating needle in (a) stiff PVC rubber with $E = 33$ kPa (b) soft PVC rubber with $E = 8.6$ kPa (c) *ex vivo* bovine liver sample, and (d) segmented needle shape from an insertion into stiff PVC with vibration at 2.6 kHz. The blue crosses indicate the needle cross sections detected using Doppler, the red line is the polynomial curve fit to the points.

3   Results

For the repeated manual test segmentations, the standard distance deviation, S_{XY} was calculated as

$$S_{XY} = \sqrt{\sum_{i=1}^{N} \frac{(d_{i,MC})^2}{N-2}}, \tag{1}$$

where $d_{i,MC}$ is the distance in the image plane between one manually selected needle point and the corresponding mean center, and N is the number of points. The standard distance deviation was 0.68 mm in the stiff PVC rubber, 0.79 mm in the soft PVC rubber, and 0.58 mm in the *ex vivo* liver tissue.

Figure 3 shows example power Doppler images of the vibrating needle in the three tissue simulants, as well as an example segmentation. The stiff PVC rubber in general showed a more concentrated Doppler response, presumably because there was less movement of the surrounding tissue. The soft PVC rubber showed a larger Doppler response than the other two tissue simulants.

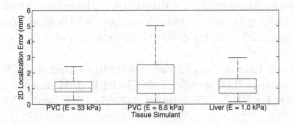

Fig. 4. Segmentation error by tissue simulant. Each tissue was tested with four different vibration frequencies, with PRF at 1666 Hz in each case. For each group, red line indicates median error, blue box indicates 25th and 75th percentile errors, whiskers indicate minimum and maximum errors.

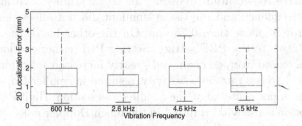

Fig. 5. Segmentation error by vibration frequency. Each vibration frequency was tested with three different tissue simulants, with PRF at 1666 Hz in each case. For each group, red line indicates median error, blue box indicates 25th and 75th percentile errors, whiskers indicate minimum and maximum errors.

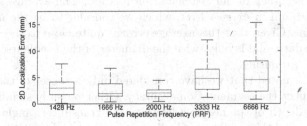

Fig. 6. Segmentation error by Doppler PRF. All tests were performed in PVC rubber with $E = 8.6$ kPa, with vibration at 2600 Hz. For each group, red line indicates median error, blue box indicates 25th and 75th percentile errors, whiskers indicate minimum and maximum errors.

Figure 4 shows a comparison of localization error based on tissue simulant. The soft PVC rubber had the highest average and maximum errors, which follows from the typical Doppler responses seen in Figure 3. The average localization errors were 1.03 mm in stiff PVC rubber, 1.24 mm in soft PVC rubber, and 1.09 mm in *ex vivo* liver.

Figure 5 shows a comparison of localization error based on vibration frequency. The average localization errors were 0.99 mm for 600 Hz vibration, 1.05 mm for 2600 Hz vibration, 1.25 mm for 4600 Hz vibration, and 1.03 mm for 6500 Hz vibration.

Figure 6 shows a comparison of localization error based on PRF. The average localization errors were 3.00 mm for 1428 Hz PRF, 1.94 mm for 1666 Hz PRF, 2.04 mm for 2000 Hz PRF, 4.75 mm for 3333 Hz PRF, and 4.50 mm for 6666 Hz PRF.

4   Discussion

The results presented in the previous section suggest that our method is not strongly sensitive to vibration frequency or tissue stiffness. Variations in both the vibration frequency and the tissue simulant did not affect the average segmentation error by more than 0.25 mm. On the other hand, the segmentation error was sensitive to the PRF setting. Setting PRF either too low or too high resulted in increased average error and greatly increased maximum error. Low PRF, equivalent to less motion sensitivity, resulted in smaller Doppler responses which were often not centered at the needle cross section. High PRF, equivalent to greater motion sensitivity, resulted in too much Doppler noise, which made it difficult to identify the needle cross section using our simple analysis technique. We hypothesize that it will be possible to optimally select the PRF setting for a specific combination of needle, tissue and vibration frequency, although the presence of blood vessels may complicate this in some clinical applications.

Without identifying a specific clinical application, it is difficult to usefully evaluate the accuracy of our segmentation method. The average segmentation error was 1.09 mm in *ex vivo* liver, which we consider to be the most realistic tissue simulant. Given that this average error is quite close to the variability in our reference data, and is only twice the diameter of the needle itself, this result appears quite promising.

It should be noted that we have considered only a subset of the parameters that might affect the segmentation accuracy. Other possibly significant parameters include depth of the needle relative to the transducer, angle between the imaging plane and the needle, needle diameter or material, and vibration amplitude.

Compared to previously described segmentation methods, our approach has the advantage that it is computationally simple. On average, the software took 32 ms to process each image when running in Matlab on a typical PC. With implementation in C++, our algorithm should easily be able to localize the needle in each 2D image during the latent time between frame captures. Typical image capture rate in our experiment was 13 frames per second, although this depends on imaging depth and size of Doppler box.

Although the piezoelectric buzzers produced sufficient motion of the needle to yield a Doppler response, the amplitude of vibration was on the order of a needle diameter in free space (approximately 0.5 mm), and likely much smaller in tissue. As a result, we believe the vibration presents a minimal safety risk to the patient; however, further investigation of this issue is needed.

One disadvantage of our method is the audible tones generated by the piezo-electric buzzers. All the vibration frequencies in this initial study were within the human audible range, and were generally loud enough to be unpleasant but not loud enough to necessitate hearing protection. We do not believe this is critical, as it should be possible to use shielding to greatly reduce the volume of noise heard by clinical staff. It might be possible to vibrate the needle just above the human audible range using a piezoelectric transducer. We are also currently exploring other actuators, such as voice coils, that should produce less audible noise.

5 Conclusion

We have described a method for using high-frequency vibration and 3D ultra-sound Doppler imaging to segment curved needles in tissue. We have demon-strated that this method results in an average error of approximately 1 to 2 mm across a range of tissue properties and vibration frequencies. In future work, we will implement this method in real-time software, and integrate it with a robotic platform in order to validate its usefulness in needle steering tasks.

References

1. Aboofazeli, M., Abolmaesumi, P., Mousavi, P., Fichtinger, G.: A new scheme for curved needle segmentation in three-dimensional ultrasound images. In: IEEE Int. Symp. Biomedical Imaging: Nano to Macro, pp. 1067–1070 (2009)
2. Armstrong, G., Cardon, L., Vlkomerson, D., Lipson, D., Wong, J., Rodriguez, L.L., Thomas, J.D., Griffin, B.P.: Localization of needle tip with color doppler during pericardiocentesis: In vitro validation and initial clinical application. J. American Soc. Echocardiography 14, 29–37 (2001)
3. Ayvaci, A., Yan, P., Xu, S., Soatto, S., Kruecker, J.: Biopsy needle detection in transrectal ultrasound. Comput. Med. Imag. Grap. 35(7), 653–659 (2011)
4. Barva, M., Uhercik, M., Mari, J.M., Kybic, J., Duhamel, J.R., Liebgott, H., Hlavac, V., Cachard, C.: Parallel integral projection transform for straight electrode local-ization in 3-D ultrasound images. IEEE Trans. Ultrason. Ferroelectr. Freq. Con-trol 55(7), 1559–1569 (2008)
5. Cheung, S., Rohling, R.: Enhancement of needle visibility in ultrasound-guided percutaneous procedures. Ultrasound Med. Biol. 30(5), 617–624 (2004)
6. Cool, D.W., Gardi, L., Romagnoli, C., Saikaly, M., Izawa, J.I., Fenster, A.: Temporal-based needle segmentation algorithm for transrectal ultrasound prostate biopsy procedures. Med. Phys. 37(4), 1660–1673 (2010)
7. Ding, M., Cardinal, H.N., Fenster, A.: Automatic needle segmentation in 3D ul-trasound images using two orthogonal 2D image projections. Med. Phys. 30(2), 222–234 (2003)
8. Ding, M., Fenster, A.: A real-time biopsy needle segmentation technique using hough transform. Med. Phys. 30(8), 2222–2233 (2003)
9. Feld, R., Needleman, L., Goldberg, B.: Use of a needle-vibrating device and color doppler imaging for sonographically guided invasive procedures. Am. J. Roentgenology 168, 255–256 (1997)

10. Fronheiser, M.P., Idriss, S.F., Wolf, P.D., Smith, S.W.: Vibrating interventional device detection using real-time 3-D color doppler. IEEE Trans. Ultrason. Ferroelectr. Freq. Control 55(6), 1355–1362 (2008)
11. Harmat, A., Rohling, R.N., Salcudean, S.E.: Needle tip localization using stylet vibration. Ultrasound Med. Biol. 32(9), 1339–1348 (2006)
12. Holen, J., Waag, R.C., Gramiak, R.: Improved needle-tip visualization by color Doppler sonography. Am. J. Roentgenol. 156, 401–402 (1985)
13. Holen, J., Waag, R.C., Gramiak, R.: Representations of rapidly oscillating structures on the Doppler display. Ultrasound Med. Biol. 11(2), 267–272 (1985)
14. Majewicz, A., Wedlick, T., Reed, K., Okamura, A.: Evaluation of robotic needle steering in ex vivo tissue. In: IEEE Int. Conf. Robotics Automation, pp. 2068–2073 (2010)
15. McAleavey, S.A., Rubens, D.J., Parker, K.J.: Doppler ultrasound imaging of magnetically vibrated brachytherapy seeds. IEEE Trans. Biomed. Eng. 50(2), 252–255 (2003)
16. Neshat, H.R.S., Patel, R.V.: Real-time parametric curved needle segmentation in 3D ultrasound images. In: IEEE RAS EMBS Int. Conf. Biomedical Robotics Biomechatronics, pp. 670–675 (2008)
17. Novotny, P.M., Stoll, J.A., Vasilyev, N.V., del Nido, P.J., Dupont, P.E., Zickler, T.E., Howe, R.D.: GPU based real-time instrument tracking with three-dimensional ultrasound. Med. Im. Anal. 11(5), 458–464 (2007)
18. Okazawa, S.H., Ebrahimi, R., Chuang, J., Rohling, R.N., Salcudean, S.E.: Methods for segmenting curved needles in ultrasound images. Med. Im. Anal. 10(3), 330–342 (2006)
19. Qiu, W., Ding, M., Yuchi, M.: Needle segmentation using 3D quick randomized hough transform. In: IEEE Int. Conf. Intelligent Networks Intelligent Systems, pp. 449–452 (2008)
20. Reddy, K.E., Light, E.D., Rivera, D.J., Kisslo, J.A., Smith, S.W.: Color doppler imaging of cardiac catheters using vibrating motors. Ultrasonic Imaging 30, 247–250 (2008)
21. Reed, K.B., Majewicz, A., Kallem, V., Alterovitz, R., Goldberg, K., Cowan, N.J., Okamura, A.M.: Robot-assisted needle steering. IEEE Robot. Autom. Mag. 18(4), 33–46 (2011)
22. Rogers, A.J., Light, E.D., Smith, S.W.: 3-D ultrasound guidance of autonomous robot for location of ferrous shrapnel. IEEE Trans. Ultrason. Ferroelectr. Freq. Control 56(7), 1301–1303 (2009)
23. Uhercík, M., Kybic, J., Liebgott, H., Cachard, C.: Model fitting using ransac for surgical tool localization in 3D ultrasound images. IEEE Trans. Biomed. Eng. 57(8), 1907–1916 (2010)
24. Wedlick, T.: Models and techniques to enhance the accuracy of robotic needle insertion. Ph.D. thesis, The Johns Hopkins University (2013)
25. Wei, Z., Gardi, L., Downey, D.B., Fenster, A.: Oblique needle segmentation and tracking for 3D TRUS guided prostate brachytherapy. Med. Phys. 32(9), 2928–2941 (2005)
26. Wood, N.A., Shahrour, K., Ost, M.C., Riviere, C.N.: Needle steering system using duty-cycled rotation for percutaneous kidney access. In: Int. Conf. IEEE EMBS, pp. 5432–5435 (2010)
27. Zhou, H., Qiu, W., Ding, M., Songgen, Z.: Automatic needle segmentation in 3D ultrasound images using 3D improved hough transform. In: SPIE Medical Imaging: Image-Guided Procedures Modeling, vol. 6918, pp. 691821-1–691821-9 (2008)

Mobile EM Field Generator for Ultrasound Guided Navigated Needle Insertions

Keno März[1], Alfred M. Franz[1], Bram Stieltjes[2], Justin Iszatt[1],
Alexander Seitel[1], Boris Radeleff[3], Hans-Peter Meinzer[1],
and Lena Maier-Hein[1]

[1] Div. of Medical and Biological Informatics, Subdivision Computer-assisted
Interventions, DKFZ Heidelberg, Germany
[2] Quantitative Imaging-based Disease Characterization, DKFZ Heidelberg, Germany
[3] Dept. of Diagnostic and Interventional Radiology, University Hospital Heidelberg
{k.maerz,l.maier-hein}@dkfz-heidelberg.de
http://www.dkfz.de

Abstract. Needle insertions are an elementary tool for diagnostic and
therapeutic purposes. Critical success factors are: Precise needle placement, avoidance of critical structures and short intervention time. Navigation solutions for ultrasound-based needle insertions have been presented but did not find widespread clinical application. This can be attributed to the complexity and higher costs introduced by additional
tracking related equipment. Using a new compact electromagnetic (EM)
field generator (FG), we present the first navigated intervention method
that combines field generator and ultrasound (US) probe into a single
mobile imaging modality that enables tracking of needle and patient. In
a phantom study, we applied the system for navigated needle insertion
and achieving a hit rate of 92% and a mean accuracy of $3.1mm$ (n=24).
These results demonstrate the potential of the new combined modality
in facilitating US-guided needle insertion.

Keywords: Electromagnetic Tracking, Computer-assisted Interventions,
Needle Insertion, Ultrasound, Liver, Biopsy, Mobile Field Generator.

1 Introduction

Needle insertions in the liver today are usually conducted under either ultrasound (US) or computed tomography (CT) guidance. In contrast to CT, US
features low costs and high availability, is easy and quick to apply, acquires
images in real-time and does not expose the patient to radiation. [1] However,
image quality suffers if adverse factors are present. Adiposity for example reduces
image contrast in the target region significantly and impedes reliable structure
identification. Furthermore, conventional needle insertions are usually performed
in-plane with a special needle guide attached to the probe that leads the needle
exactly along the ultrasound plane. This way, it is assured that the needle is is
always visible in the US image. Linking needle and probe leads to a decreased

D. Barratt et al. (Eds.): IPCAI 2013, LNCS 7915, pp. 71–80, 2013.

flexibility, as the probe can hardly be moved during the needle insertion. Nevertheless, it is often necessary to use a needle guide as the cross section of a needle is very small and hard to discern in an ultrasound image. This in turn makes it hard to determine the trajectory of the needle correctly when working extraplane. If critical structures are situated along the needle insertion trajectory, the procedure is complicated further. In case the physician decides that the needle insertion is too risky or complicated under ultrasound guidance, it will usually be performed under CT guidance[2], incurring additional costs and exposition to radiation through several CT scans.

The majority of needle insertions in the liver are performed under US-guidance. [3] Especially when needle insertion trajectories are short and already traverse in a safe distance to critical structures the needle insertion can easily be performed under US guidance and neither CT-based approaches nor navigation support would be beneficial in these cases. However, in more complicated cases, where even CT-guided needle insertions are challenging, a navigated US-guidance would improve the procedure, providing both real-time imaging and tracking of the instrument. Accordingly, the goal of a navigated US-guided needle insertion system should be to assist the physician in complex situations and thus enable him to perform needle insertions under US-guidance, where he would have resorted to CT-guidance before.

To allow US-guided insertions in complex situations, navigation solutions have been proposed by various authors and companies like Ultrasonix and General Electrics.[4][5][6][7] However, they usually require preoperative data or the usage of additional modalities. This complicates the technically uncomplex workflow of an US-guided needle insertion and impedes adoption into the clinical workflow. As a result, these systems have not found widespread clinical application. Most navigation solutions use tracking technology to localize instruments and patients. This is typically achieved with optical or electromagnetic (EM) tracking systems. EM tracking systems offer the advantage of not requiring a line of sight to the tracked objects. Thus, they are able to directly track the needle tip, which avoids tracking errors trough needle bending and allows the usage of thinner needles, thereby reducing invasivity. As stated by Maier-Hein *et al.*, two of the main challenges associated with EM tracking are the compensation of systematic distance errors arising from the influence of metal near the field generator (FG) and the optimized setup of the FG to maximize tracking accuracy in the area of interest. [8] To address these issues, a new mobile and compact FG (NDI Aurora® *Compact FG 7-10*, see Fig.1b) has recently been presented by NDI (NorthernDigital Inc.,Waterloo, Canada). Studies have shown that the new FG is less susceptible to interference than former models. [8] Furthermore, interference caused by connecting US probes to it is negligible. [9] Moving the FG together with the probe implies high precision and accuracy, since the area of interest automatically and continuously is situated near the center of the tracking volume. At the same time, it keeps the FG away from typical sources of interference like metallic patient stretchers.

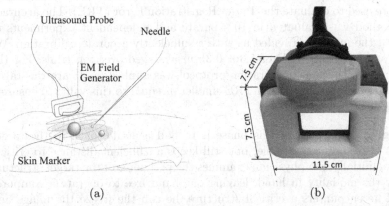

Fig. 1. (a) The setup of the navigation solution. (b) Compact field generator and US probe combined into a prototype modality. The large curved array type US probe did not fit trough the central hole and was mounted on the side. The complete setup weighed 200g of which the FG contributed 100g.

We use the compact FG attached to an US-Probe as a mobile imaging modality that allows to locate EM-tracked instruments directly (See Fig.1b). In this study, we present a new navigation solution in which we apply this combined modality in a navigation solution and evaluate it in a phantom study.

2   Material and Methods

The Field Generator was combined into a single modality with the US probe as shown in Fig.1b. The FG has a central opening that would theoretically make it possible to mount a US probe in it. However, needle insertions into the liver usually are performed using relatively large curved array probes that do not fit trough the opening. The far cable end sockets are too large as well, requiring us to use the shown side mount for our experimental prototype. Nevertheless, the usage of the central mount has been evaluated experimentally. [9] Combining FG and US Probe has the implication of permanently placing the US image plane in the tracking volume as both move in unison. The complete setup is shown in Fig.1a. Additionally, as a means of tracking the patient, a skin marker is attached close to the lesion thus allowing the tracking of critical structures in 3D.

Calibration: To calibrate the probe against the FG we performed a simple point based calibration following Muratore and Galloway[10], which did not require additional hardware and can quickly be performed by a single person in a couple of minutes. 22 needle insertions were performed in a gelatin phantom and the tip, once visible in the US image, was marked manually. The pattern encompassed the whole US image plane. 13 Points where used for calibration, the remaining 9 points were used to evaluate the Target Registration Error (TRE). The accuracy of this method was evaluated in 10 separate and independent experiments to assure that the method provided us with a sufficiently accurate calibration. We achieved a mean RMS TRE of $1.3 \pm 0.3mm$ averaged over ten trials. For the phantom study, the same calibration protocol was applied, and care was taken to only allow calibrations with a TRE smaller or equal to this value to ensure a basic quality of registration.

Planning: The purpose of this phase is to find a needle path to the target zone that is as short as possible, but still keeps a sufficient distance to critical structures. Initially, the physician examines the perimeter of the target structure with only the modality in hand, leaving one hand free to operate a computer mouse. If he encounters a critical structure, he can the freeze the image and mark the structure on it. A sphere around the structure appears, marking the area as a critical zone. These critical zone includes the critical structure (e.g. the vena portae) that must not be harmed and a safety margin around it, the size of which is at the physician's discretion. Although shapes other than spheres can be placed, we consciously limited ourselves to spheres for this evaluation, as they are easy to handle for the user and other structures can quickly be approximated by placing a series of spheres. To tell different zones apart, they can be assigned colors and labels. The pose of the zones during the intervention is continuously tracked relatively to the skin marker under a rigid body assumption. Accordingly, assessment of both the needle's and the US image's pose in relation to the target structure and critical zones is possible at any time. When the physician is content with the zone placement, he positions the needle's tip on the skin and starts the navigation.

Navigation: The system helps the physician guide the needle to the target zone using the guidance view shown in Fig.2. It projects the path of the needle onto the image plane, which has been shown to be a helpful feature.[7] Additionally a 3D scene is shown, in which the US image, the needle and the critical structures are rendered. The 3D scene can be switched between a view from the tip of the needle along the needle axis and a free fly view. The former allows for exact navigation past critical zones, the latter gives a clear overview of the intervention area. For each zone, a bar is shown that visualizes the distance to the zone, providing visual feedback if the needle tip approaches a zone and turning red if the distance falls below a definable value. These auxiliary means enable the physician to assess the state of the intervention at any time.

2.1   Evaluation

To prototype the navigation solution, we used the Medical Imaging and Interaction Toolkit (MITK, *www.mitk.org*) [11] since it offers image manipulation tools and supports tracking via the Image Guided Therapy (IGT) Module [12].

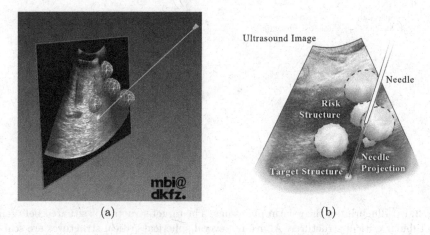

(a)   (b)

Fig. 2. (a) Screenshot of the navigation view with critical structures inside as well as in front of and behind the image plane. (b) Corresponding illustration.

To evaluate our navigational approach, nine identical phantoms representing high critical situations were manufactured using ballistic gelatin (GELITA AG, Eberbach, Germany)(See Fig.3b). The gelatin used mimics the properties of human tissue. The target structure was situated to be hard to reach without violating a critical structure (see Fig.3a). The target was placed between two tubular critical structures, with several spherical critical structures spread out above it. One structure in particular was always present directly above the target. The upper layer of critical structures lay between 6 to 7 cm deep, with the target lying at a depth of 9 to 10 cm. Finally, a layer of gelatin containing black color was applied on top of the phantom to prevent direct sight onto the insertion area. A physician and a technician performed 14 needle insertions each, the first two of which were not evaluated and regarded as practice runs.

3   Results

Table 1 shows the results of the phantom study. Two critical structures were violated, which in both cases had not been marked. Physician and technician achieved an accuracy of $2.8mm$ and $3.4mm$ respectively and both missed the target one time resulting in a hit rate of 92%. The physician later stated that his miss of the target structure was a result of him trying to manually correct the needle's position, which resulted in the miss. In this case, the software showed that the structure was missed.

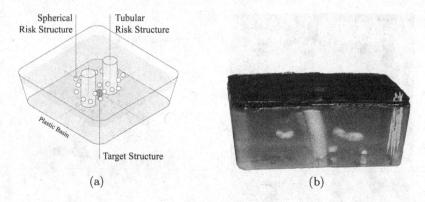

Fig. 3. (a) Blueprint of the gelatin phantoms. The target structure is situated between two tubular critical structures. Above it, several spherical critical structures are scattered. (b) The finished phantom where tubular and spherical critical structures are clearly visible.

4   Discussion

Solutions for navigated US-guided needle insertions have yet been unable to achieve widespread clinical application. An important factor for this seems to be the added complexity that negates one of biggest advantages of US: Its quick and relatively simple application. To our knowledge, this is the first approach to combine an ultrasound probe with a compact field generator and integrate this new modality into a navigation solution. The results are promising. The mean accuracy of $3.1 \pm 1.2mm$ is in the same range as previous approaches. Comparable experiments in CT-guided marker-based approaches achieved mean accuracies of $2.7 \pm 0.7mm$ using EM Tracking in gelatin phantoms [13] and $3.7 \pm 2.3mm$ using optical tracking in an in-vivo porcine liver. [2] We decided against a direct comparison of conventional in-plane versus our navigation approach as we do not intend to replace the conventional approach. When the situation allows it due to low complexity, a physician will mostly prefer the unnavigated approach over a more complex navigated one. However, we intend to make needle insertions under US guidance possible where before a CT-guided approach was required. Our solution enables the physician to keep his workflow while giving him a range of options and aids if necessary. By establishing and tracking critical zones, lesions that are difficult to access can be reached more safely. Since the FG is linked with the probe, the tracking volume is relatively far away from metallic components compared to classical EM FGs. This makes the system robust against interference from metallic or ferromagnetic objects such as a patient stretcher. [8]

Calibration of US images with tracking systems is a much discussed subject. Several calibration solutions have been presented in literature. Besides point based approaches, Cross-Wire and N-Wire phantom techniques are widespread

Table 1. Results of the phantom study. Measured parameters were the percentage of insertions that hit the target (*Hit Rate*), the distance between needle tip and target center (*Accuracy*), the number of violated critical structures (*Violations*), the minimal distance between needle and the nearest critical structures surface (*Margin*), the number of partial or total needle retractions (*Retractions*) and the length of the procedure from the time the needle first penetrated the phantom's surface to the time the physician declared the target hit (*Duration*). The latter three parameters were acquired by performing a control CT scan of each phantom after the needle insertion.

	Physician	Technician	Total
n	12	12	24
Hit Rate	92%	92%	92%
Accuracy	$2.8 \pm 1.1mm$	$3.4 \pm 1.2mm$	$3.1 \pm 1.2mm$
Violations	2	0	2
Margin	$4.6 \pm 3.3mm$	$9.0 \pm 4.5mm$	$4.6 \pm 3.9mm$
Retractions	0.8 ± 0.6	0.9 ± 0.8	0.9 ± 0.7
Duration	$82 \pm 39s$	$42 \pm 21s$	$62 \pm 30s$

means of calibration. [14] We favored a simple approach[10], but still achieved a surprisingly good TRE of $1.3mm$. A possible explanation could be the beneficial effects of having a fixed transformation between image plane and tracking volume, further research could provide insight in this matter. An additional effect of this setup is that the needle automatically is placed near the center of the field into the area of highest accuracy. In traditional setups, constant field shifts are eliminated by subtracting the reported coordinates of the transducer from those of the needle. This applies to our risk structure tracking as well, as they are being localized by using the attached sensor. However, our results do not indicate significant errors. This can be explained by the fact that the instruments are so close to the FG that the first order shifts are relatively small and the fact that we only need one transformation and accordingly only have one dynamic source of error for the needle to image transformation.

It was originally planned to perform 15 needle insertions plus two practice insertions by each a physician with ultrasound guided needle insertion experience and by a technician without such experience. However, the targets randomly drew air after needle insertion, impeding visibility in the US image and rendering some of them unusable for further experiments. As a result, only 14 needle insertions including the two test runs could be performed. For future experiments, we suggest to use multiple targets if more than one needle insertion is planned.

The results show that critical structure can safely be avoided when they are correctly marked. Both of the violated structures were hit because they have not been marked. The hit rate can be regarded as good, with one miss each. In one case, the system predicted the miss correctly. This is comparable to previous experiments by Sindram *et al.* with an US guided navigation system using optical tracking, where a total hit rate of 88% was achieved. [7] During the experiments the 21G needles bent significantly in the ballistic gelatin (see Fig.4). This made

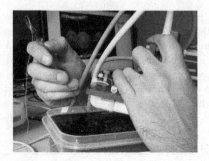

Fig. 4. Navigated US-guided needle insertion into a gel phantom. Note the needle and the field generator directly above its entry point.

corrections of the trajectory necessary several times. Still, both physician and technician retracted the needle less than once per needle insertion on average. For this study, we decided to not mark the target structure but instead use the ultrasound probe to follow it. This seems preferable: Since the US-image is always current, breathing motions can be observed in real time. Critical areas should however always be marked and are usually placed with a considerable security margin. This makes them less susceptible to errors in motion compensation, as the physicians goal is to stay clear of them by a wide margin.

The technician showed a shorter mean time for insertion duration, which seems surprising. This can be explained with the technician trusting the system blindly while the physician, using his experience, took care to evaluate the US image. The technician put the needle on the phantoms surface, used the projection to gauge the trajectory and then quickly moved the needle forward, correcting the needle's path based on the projection. The physician on the other hand carefully advanced the needle and used the US probe to validate the trajectory.

Regarding the handling of the modality, it would be beneficial to be able to use the central mounting hole. Mounting the field generator on the side of the probe extends the available tracking volume in one direction, which increases the available space for needle handling. On the other hand, the modality becomes more unwieldy, restricting probe pitch and requiring the physician to use a relatively steep angle for the probe pose. This problem is solvable when producing probes that have an internal field generator. The setup adds a weight of approximately 200g to the probe and increases it's size by 7.5 cm in depth and brings the complete modality to 11.5 cm in width. The added width seems negligible as probes are wide by nature, however the added depth requires the physician to adjust his grip a little to the rear end of the probe, where he can then hold it naturally. Finding a more ergonomic form and optimizing weight is another problem that can be solved with direct integration and the authors believe that handling a combined modality is a matter of habit. It has been shown that normal probes do not interfere with the EM field in a significant manner[9], however this has not been verified for motorized US probes. Nevertheless, these transducers play a relatively minor role in abdominal needle insertions.

Future work comprises e.g. semiautomatic segmentation methods, which could speed up planning and provide a more direct visual feedback on the zones nature. Motion compensation is another interesting topic which could improve critical structure avoidance. [15] Path planning approaches could help in highly difficult situations where only narrow safe canals lead to the target. [16] We evaluated our navigation system in a rigid phantom study. US-guided needle insertions are usually performed under respiratory pause ("holding breath"). Still, the system should be evaluated in a more realistic setting under respiratory motion. The study has not been executed in an operating room. However, US guided needle insertions do not require specific rooms as for example a CT guided approach does, where the metallic patient stretcher poses significant problems. [2] Further-more, a careful evaluation regarding commercial systems would be of benefit.

In conclusion our results show that our approach is accurate with a mean targeting error of $3.1mm$. Combining the field generator with the ultrasound probe solves a number of problems like the positioning of the generator and interference elegantly while allowing the physician to keep his workflow. These results clearly show the potential of the new FG as a replacement for current field generators and the authors believe that a combined modality will help US navigation approaches to transition into clinical workflows on a larger scale.

Acknowledgments. This study was conducted with support of the "Research Training Group 1126: Intelligent Surgery" funded by the German Research Foun-dation (DFG). The authors would like to thank Sigmar Fröhlich, Gina Jackson, Stefan Kirsch and Nina Stecker (NDI Europe GmbH) for providing additional needles for the experiment.

References

1. Khati, N.J., Gorodenker, J., Hill, M.: Ultrasound-Guided Biopsies of the Abdomen. Ultrasound Quartely 27(4), 255–268 (2011)
2. Maier-Hein, L., Tekbas, A., Seitel, A., Pianka, F., Müller, S.A., Satzl, S., et al.: In vivo accuracy assessment of a needle-based navigation system for CT-guided radiofrequency ablation of the liver. Medical Physics 35(12), 5385–5396 (2008)
3. Kliewer, M.A., Sheafor, D.H., Paulson, E.K., Helsper, R.S., Hertzberg, B.S., Nel-son, R.C.: Percutaneous Liver Biopsy: a Cost-Benefit Analysis Comparing Sono-graphic and CT Guidance. American Journal of Roentgenology 173(5), 1199–1202 (1999)
4. Clevert, D.A., Paprottka, P.M., Helck, A., Reiser, M., Trumm, C.G.: Image fusion in the management of thermal tumor ablation of the liver. Clinical Hemorheology and Microcirculation (September 2012) (epub ahead of print)
5. Noble, J.A., Boukerroui, D.: Ultrasound Image Segmentation: A Survey. IEEE Transactions on Medical Imaging 25(8), 987–1010 (2006)
6. Solberg, O.V., Lindseth, F., Torp, H., Blake, R.E., Hernes, T.A.N.: Freehand 3D Ultrasound Reconstruction Algorithms – A Review. Ultrasound in Medicine and Biology 33(7), 991–1009 (2007)

7. Sindram, D., Swan, R.Z., Lau, K.N., McKillop, I.H., Iannitti, D.A., Martinie, J.B.: Real-time three-dimensional guided ultrasound targeting system for microwave ablation of liver tumours: a human pilot study. HPB 13(3), 185–191 (2011)
8. Maier-Hein, L., Franz, A.M., Birkfellner, W., Hummel, J., Gergel, I., Wegner, I., et al.: Standardized assessment of new electromagnetic field generators in an interventional radiology setting. Medical Physics 39(6), 3424–3434 (2012)
9. Franz, A.M., März, K., Hummel, J., Birkfellner, W., Bendl, R., Delorme, S., et al.: Electromagnetic tracking for US-guided interventions: standardized assessment of a new compact field generator. International Journal of Computer Assisted Radiology and Surgery 7(6), 813–818 (2012)
10. Muratore, D.M., Galloway, R.L.: Beam calibration without a phantom for creating a 3-D freehand ultrasound system. Ultrasound in Medicine and Biology 27(11), 1557–1566 (2001)
11. Wolf, I., Vetter, M., Wegner, I., Böttger, T., Nolden, M., Schöbinger, M., et al.: The medical imaging interaction toolkit. Medical Image Analysis 9(6), 594–604 (2005)
12. Neuhaus, J., Wegner, I., Kast, J., Baumhauer, M., Seitel, A., Gergel, I., et al.: MITK-IGT: Eine Navigationskomponente für das Medical Imaging Interaction Toolkit. In: Tagungsband der BVM 2009, pp. 454–458 (2009)
13. Franz, A.M., Servatius, M., Seitel, A., Kauczor, H.U., Meinzer, H.P., Maier-Hein, L.: Navigated targeting of liver lesions: pitfalls of electromagnetic tracking. Biomedical Engineering 57(1), 897–900 (2008)
14. Mercier, L., Lang, T., Lindseth, F., Collins, D.L.: A review of calibration techniques for freehand 3-D ultrasound systems. Ultrasound in Medicine and Biology 31(4), 449–471 (2005)
15. McClelland, J.R., Hawkes, D.J., Schaeffter, T., King, A.P.: Respiratory Motion Models: A Review. Medical Image Analysis 17(1), 19–42 (2013)
16. Seitel, A., Engel, M., Sommer, C.M., Radeleff, B.A., Essert-Villard, C., Baegert, C., et al.: Computer-Assisted Trajectory Planning for Percutaneous Needle Insertions. Med. Phys. 38(6), 3246–3259 (2011)

First Flexible Robotic Intra-operative Nuclear Imaging for Image-Guided Surgery

José Gardiazabal[1,2], Tobias Reichl[1], Aslı Okur[1,2],
Tobias Lasser[1,3], and Nassir Navab[1]

[1] Computer Aided Medical Procedures, Technische Universität München, Germany
[2] Department of Nuclear Medicine, Klinikum rechts der Isar,
Technische Universität München, Germany
[3] Institute of Biomathematics and Biometry, Helmholtz Zentrum München, Germany
gardiaza@cs.tum.edu

Abstract. Functional imaging systems for intra-operative use, like free-hand SPECT, have been successfully demonstrated in the past, with remarkable results. These results, even though very positive in some cases, tend to suffer from high variability depending on the expertise of the operator. A well trained operator can produce datasets that will lead to a reconstruction that can rival a conventional SPECT machine, while an untrained one will not be able to achieve such results. In this paper we present a flexible robotic functional nuclear imaging setup for intra-operative use, replacing the operator in the scanning process with a robotic arm. The robot can assure good coverage of the area of interest, thus producing a consistent scanning pattern that can be reproduced with high accuracy, and provides the option to compensate for radioactive decay. We show first results on phantoms demonstrating the feasibility of the setup to perform 3D nuclear imaging suitable for the operating room.

1 Introduction

Functional nuclear imaging modalities like PET or SPECT have traditionally been used for cancer diagnosis [1]. By injecting a radioactive tracer and acquiring data of the patient inside the imaging device, a 3D image of the distribution of radioactivity inside the body is reconstructed. The achievable resolution of 4–8 mm makes it a suitable for diagnosis. Moving to the operating room however, the size and weight of the devices are prohibitive, a large part of which is due to the detectors and collimators.

To acquire functional information intra-operatively, a common solution is thus to use hand-held single pixel gamma detectors. They work like a Geiger counter, emitting a sound which changes according to the radiation detected. Those are directionally collimated, so the surgeon is able to narrow down from where the radiation is coming. For 3D intra-operative imaging, a method called Freehand SPECT was proposed [2], combining a gamma detector with an optical tracking system to enable tomographic reconstruction of a SPECT-like image by manually

D. Barratt et al. (Eds.): IPCAI 2013, LNCS 7915, pp. 81–90, 2013.
© Springer-Verlag Berlin Heidelberg 2013

scanning around the area of interest. It has been shown [3] that the main defining factor of the method's image quality is the quality of the scanning trajectory, which leads to experienced users performing systematically better than novice ones. Due to the freehand nature of the scan it is also impossible to exactly reproduce a scan. These two issues limit the practical usefulness of the Freehand SPECT method in clinical practice.

To address these issues, the scanning trajectory has to be optimized and to be of a guaranteed sufficient quality. While training the surgeons and providing visual guidance to the surgeons significantly improves quality [4], reproducibility remains an issue. This is our motivation for suggesting to support the surgeon with a robotic arm that is capable of scanning in a fully- or semi-automated fashion. This will provide results that are fully operator independent, but will also allow custom-optimized trajectories with sufficient coverage of the region of interest, while guaranteeing highly reproducible scans, for example before, during, and after surgery. Additionally, the ability to control the scanning speed enables compensation for radioactive decay, to ensure reproducible detection statistics.

While this will mark, to our knowledge, the first fully flexible intra-operative functional imaging setup, other robotic systems have already been presented for intra-operative imaging. One major example is for regular [5] and transrectal ultrasound imaging [6]. While these systems aim at 3D imaging, no tomographic reconstruction is needed, and thus the trajectories are far less complex than for nuclear tomographic imaging, and the reconstructed image is not as operator-dependent. Another example is the case of robotic measurement of oxygen tension in mice [7], where the robot is used to position the oxygen probes, and the challenge is to keep the probes in the correct area. Similarly, the "Artis zeego" X-ray C-arm (Siemens Healthcare, Erlangen, Germany) employs a flexible robotic arm, but still follows a standard C-arm imaging protocol with 180 degrees (or more) angular coverage.

In the following we will present a fully flexible robotic system for intra-operative nuclear imaging. We will demonstrate through phantom experiments that it can match human scanning trajectories, guarantee reproducibility, and can compensate for radioactive decay.

2   Setup and Methods

Our setup consists of a six-axis robot arm (UR-6-85-5-A, Universal Robots, Odense, Denmark) holding a gamma detector (HiSens, Crystal Photonics, Berlin, Germany) with their 60°collimator for radioactivity measurements. In order to determine the position of the gamma detector relative to the region of interest, an optical tracking system (Polaris Vicra, Northern Digital, Waterloo, ON, Canada) is used with tracking targets mounted on the phantom and the gamma detector. The setup is shown in Fig. 1.

Calibration. The spatial relation between the gamma detector tip and the tracking target was determined using a custom-made cylindrical calibrator tightly

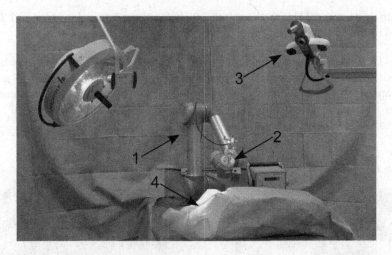

Fig. 1. Experimental setup showing the (1) robotic arm, (2) gamma detector, (3) optical tracking system and (4) phantom

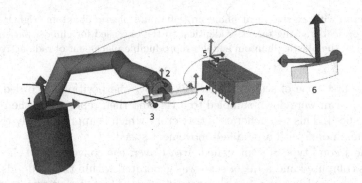

Fig. 2. Coordinate systems: (1) robot base, (2) robot hand, (3) detector target, (4) detector tip, (5) phantom target and (6) optical tracking system. All transformations can either be pre-calibrated (detector calibration, hand-eye calibration), measured intra-operatively (robot, optical tracking system), or computed from others.

fitting around the detector, while the location of the detector crystal within the detector is known by construction. The relation between tracking target and robot hand was determined fully automatically using hand-eye calibration [8]. Thus, the relation between the detection crystal and the robot hand can be computed. Fig. 2 shows the different coordinate systems involved.

Data Acquisition. During the scan, time stamps, gamma detector measurements, and detector tip position and orientation were recorded. For positioning, measurements were used either from the optical tracking system (for scans done by humans), or from the robot (for robotic scans due to the higher precision). The sampling rate was 60 Hz for the robot, 60 Hz for the gamma detector, and 20 Hz for the optical tracking system.

Robot Trajectories. Two phantoms were scanned during the experiments, an ex-vivo meat phantom and a plastic phantom, see Fig. 3. In order to generate scanning trajectories for the ex-vivo meat phantom, it was first scanned by human operators. These scans were then used to generate two types of robot trajectories:

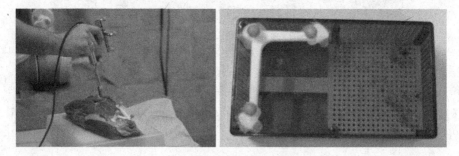

Fig. 3. Setup with ex-vivo meat phantom (left), and plastic phantom (right). In both cases the optical tracking target is identical to the one used for clinical patients. The hole raster of the plastic phantom enables reproducible placement of radioactive seeds.

For the first type of scan, called *Path Follow*, the positions recorded during the human scan were down-sampled to 5 Hz, and then replayed by the robot at constant speed. This will generate a trajectory which is approximately the same as the human one, with a modified movement speed.

For the second type of scan, called *Area Cover*, the convex hull of the human path was computed and a raster scan was generated within these bounds, which was then executed by the robot at constant speed. The different trajectories can be seen in Fig. 4.

To scan the plastic phantom, since the geometry is known and regular, the scanning pattern was a basic raster scan with constant speed over three orthogonal faces of the phantom.

Decay Compensation. As radioactivity decays over time, the exposure time for each measurement has to be prolonged in order to achieve constant photon detection statistics and thus comparable image quality. This becomes particularly relevant once a half-life of the radioactive tracer (or more) has passed, which in the clinical case for the commonly used Technetium-99m (^{99m}Tc) is 6.01 hours. In this case, adjusting the acquisition speed of the robot accordingly compensates for the decay.

Reconstruction. After acquisition, the 3D activity distribution in the volume of interest was reconstructed from the recorded data, using an iterative reconstruction technique (MLEM, [4]) and custom detection models for the gamma

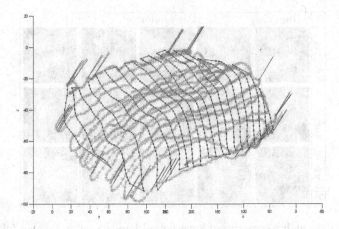

Fig. 4. Area cover scan (black crosses, view direction in red) synthesised from human input (green circles, view direction in blue). Please note that the area of interest and surface curvature only need to be roughly outlined in the human input.

detector [9]. The voxel size was 2.5 mm for the ex-vivo meat phantom and 1.5 mm for the plastic phantom. The reconstruction volumes were $17.5 \times 17.5 \times 12.5 \text{ cm}^3$ and $13.5 \times 11.25 \times 4.5 \text{ cm}^3$ respectively. The position of the probe was computed using the phantom's tracking target as reference.

3   Experiments and Results

We conducted two sets of experiments, the first set to show that robotic acquisitions can perform consistent and reproducible scans, while the second set shows the usefulness of decay compensation.

For the first set of experiments, an ex-vivo meat phantom was used, containing three radioactive seeds (1.5 mL with a solution of 1.5 MBq of ^{99m}Tc each). The phantom was scanned by three human operators, one expert and two novices, two times each. The best scan of each operator was selected, and then used to generate a path follow scan as well as an area cover scan. The path follow scan was performed by the robot three times, and the area cover scan was performed once.

Since the radioactive seeds were located at different depths, the plane containing all three hotspots was extracted from the 3D reconstruction using Principal Component Analysis (PCA) for visualisation purposes, see Fig. 5.

Fig. 6 shows an intensity profile across two hotspots for the human expert scan and for the robotic scans.

As a measure of reproducibility, the normalised cross correlation (NCC) was computed between the reconstructed volumes (summed up along the z-axis to yield a single slice) from the two repeated human and the three repeated robotic scans with the path follow trajectory, see Table 1.

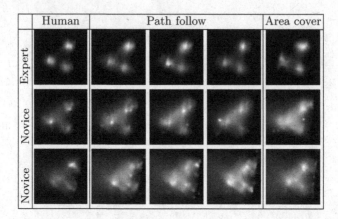

Fig. 5. Slices through reconstructed images from human operator, robot following human path (three scans), and robot following synthetic path covering area of interest

Table 1. Normalized cross correlation between two operator scans, versus the robotic scan pairs 1-2, 1-3 and 2-3 from the path follow trajectory. Reproducibility is consistently higher for reconstructions from robotic scans than for human scans.

NCC	Human 1-2	Robot 1-2	Robot 2-3	Robot 1-3
Expert	0.942	0.990	0.979	0.989
Novice	0.709	0.980	0.971	0.980
Novice	0.896	0.966	0.973	0.965

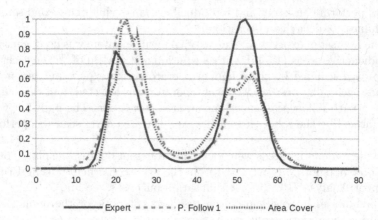

Fig. 6. Normalized intensity profiles across the rightmost two hotspots in Fig.5, for expert and robotic scans. Distance (X-axis) in mm.

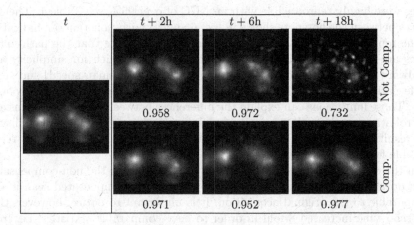

Fig. 7. Decay compensation experiment. In each column, both images were acquired at approximately the same time $t + x$. Images in upper row were acquired without decay compensation, images in lower row were acquired with decay compensation (i.e. suitably adjusted slower scanning speeds). NCC values with the image at time t are shown below each image at $t + x$. Please note the image degradation, especially in the uncompensated image at $t + 18$h.

For the second set of experiments, a plastic phantom containing three spherical seeds (250 μL with a solution of 500 kBq of ^{99m}Tc each) was used.

A raster scan over three orthogonal sides of the phantom was performed, and used as reference (time t). At $t + 2$ hours, $t + 6$ hours and $t + 18$ hours, the same scan was repeated two times each, once using the original acquisition speed, and once with reduced speed to compensate for radioactive decay. In order to evaluate the compensation, again the NCC was computed between the reconstructions at time $t + x$ and the original reconstruction at time t, see Fig. 7. The volumes were again summed up along the z-axis to yield single slices for the NCC computation.

4 Discussion

The procedure to generate SPECT images from freehand acquisitions is very challenging. Since the acquisition time is shorter and the detector area is considerably smaller, the total number of photons is considerably less than in a conventional SPECT machine. Their uses, on the other hand are very different. The SPECT machine is used for the diagnostics, and it requires a reasonably high image quality. The freehand acquisition, on the other hand are performed for guidance purposes, so the exact amplitude of the hot spots are less relevant, assuming that is possible to detect and separate them.

Fig. 5 and Fig. 6 show that robotic scans can provide image quality and hotspot separability close to a human expert operator. Furthermore, all robotic scans were highly reproducible with an NCC of over 95%, see Table 1. The distances between the hotspots shown in Fig. 6 appear fairly constant, an indication of the reproducibility of the scans. It is important to note that the path-follow scans are an approximation of the real human scan, which for simplicity and hardware limitations were not performed at the same human speed, and small angle variations during the scan were simply not reproduced my the robotic arm. Those limitations can explain the differences between the human scans and the robotic ones, but what is important to notice here is the reproducibility of the results obtained by the robot arm, as shown before, something not really possible for human operators.

In the decay compensation experiment, after 18 hours, the non-compensated scan does not yield a meaningful image, whereas the compensated scan is still comparable to the original acquisition. It is important to notice, however, that the scan time increased 8-fold in order to have comparable statistics, i.e. from 5 to 40 minutes. This is particularly important because a 40 minute scan is not feasible with human operators, but easily doable with the robotic arm. Estimation of the count rate and extrapolation is very challenging, the peak count on the first scan is 600 cps, versus 40 cps after 18 hours. This experiment is particularly relevant to the clinical workflow of our medical partners. The common procedure in sentinel lymph node biopsy for breast cancer is to inject ^{99m}Tc to the patient during noon, acquire a scintigraphy image for lymphatic mapping, and in the next morning the patient undergoes surgery. Such a decay compensation with robotic imaging can provide more reliable images for incision planning compared to the ones achieved by much shorter freehand scans.

5   Future Research

Our method for synthesizing the scan patterns is a first approach towards less dependency on a human operator, but obviously still depends on the original human scan quality. Instead, the convex hull area of the area cover scan could also be obtained from a CT image of the patient, for higher operator independence. Another option is to have the surgeon use a tracked pointer to delineate the scanning area, incorporating his expert knowledge of the area of interest.

The characteristics of a "good" scan pattern for "freehand" acquisitions are still subject of intense research [10,11]. However, complex scan patterns can hardly be communicated to humans, in particular when accurate orientation is involved, so up to now such patterns could only be evaluated in simulations. Our system now enables evaluation of such optimized scan trajectories with actual acquisition systems [11], so we expect significant mutual benefit in the future. Possible feedback loops during acquisition could also include refinement of known hotspots, or the inclusion of preliminary reconstruction results or other prior data. In the simplest case, the speed of the robot could be reduced in regions where higher activity is detected (or expected), with a quick overview scan in the beginning.

For intra-operative nuclear imaging the connection to surgical robotics is obvious: If intra-operative images are acquired in the same coordinate frame as the surgery will be performed in later, no erroneous and error-prone co-registration of images and work-spaces is needed. Intra-operatively, robots may even be used for monitoring changes and progress [12]. For this purpose, even a gamma camera may be used instead of a single-pixel detector [13], which is heavier (about 1 kilogram, versus 200 gram single detector) and thus not amenable for long-term human free-hand operation, but still feasible for a robot.

The robot used in our set-up has redundant safety features generating a protective stop if the force exceeds 150 Newtons. While this is sufficient for research and development and no additional safety guards are needed between robot and operator, for use on patients further safety measures will need to be introduced [14]. Since in our application we do not need to touch the patient, an additional distance measurement sensor could be mounted next to the gamma detector, ensuring a safe distance from the patient even in the case of errors in tracking or registration.

As with freehand SPECT, the position of the probe was always computed relative to the reference tracking target placed on the patient, e.g. on the sternum for breast cancer patients. This is the standard procedure with freehand SPECT, so the respiratory movements such as breathing are partially compensated. However, the main challenge here is that the actual acquisition and the interpretation of the images happen in different phases of the surgery, so deformations due to patient movement and anatomy changes still remain as an issue. This can be solved in the future by using additional acquisition sensors such as gamma cameras, which would allow even much faster acquisitions resulting in multiple reconstructions within the procedure.

6 Conclusion

In this work we presented the first setup for flexible robot-controlled intra-operative functional imaging with a first evaluation of its performance. This combination enables patient-specific, flexible imaging in the operating room, which easily integrates with the current surgical workflow and generates high-quality functional imaging for the guidance of surgeons. Our results are very promising in terms of accuracy, repeatability, operator-independence and medical impact, so we believe that the proposed method will lead to new applications and insights in intra-operative functional imaging.

Acknowledgments. This work was partially funded by DFG SFB824, the European Union FP7 under grant N°256984, and the TUM Graduate School of Information Science in Health (GSISH).   *

References

1. Buck, A., Nekolla, S., Ziegler, S., Beer, A., Krause, B., Herrmann, K., Scheidhauer, K., Wester, H.J., Rummeny, E., Schwaiger, M., Drzezga, A.: SPECT/CT. J. Nucl. Med. 49(8), 1305–1319 (2008)

2. Wendler, T., Hartl, A., Lasser, T., Traub, J., Daghighian, F., Ziegler, S.I., Navab, N.: Towards intra-operative 3D nuclear imaging: Reconstruction of 3D radioactive distributions using tracked gamma probes. In: Ayache, N., Ourselin, S., Maeder, A. (eds.) MICCAI 2007, Part II. LNCS, vol. 4792, pp. 909–917. Springer, Heidelberg (2007)
3. Lasser, T., Wendler, T., Ziegler, S.I., Navab, N.: Towards reproducibility of free-hand 3D tomographic nuclear imaging. In: Proceedings of IEEE Medical Imaging Conference (IEEE MIC), Dresden, Germany (October 2008)
4. Wendler, T., Herrmann, K., Schnelzer, A., Lasser, T., Traub, J., Kutter, O., Ehlerding, A., Scheidhauer, K., Schuster, T., Kiechle, M., Schwaiger, M., Navab, N., Ziegler, S.I., Buck, A.K.: First demonstration of 3-D lymphatic mapping in breast cancer using freehand SPECT. Eur. J. Nucl. Med. Mol. Imaging 37(8), 1452–1461 (2010)
5. Conti, F., Park, J., Khatib, O.: Interface design and control strategies for a robot assisted ultrasonic examination system. In: Khatib, O., Kumar, V., Sukhatme, G. (eds.) Experimental Robotics. STAR, vol. 79, pp. 97–113. Springer, Heidelberg (2012)
6. Adebar, T., Salcudean, S., Mahdavi, S., Moradi, M., Nguan, C., Goldenberg, L.: A robotic system for intra-operative trans-rectal ultrasound and ultrasound elastography in radical prostatectomy. In: Taylor, R.H., Yang, G.-Z. (eds.) IPCAI 2011. LNCS, vol. 6689, pp. 79–89. Springer, Heidelberg (2011)
7. Chang, J., Wen, B., Zanzonico, P., Kazanzides, P., Finn, R., Fichtinger, G., Ling, C.C.: A robotic system for ^{18}F–FMISO PET–guided intratumoral pO_2 measurements. Medical Physics 36(11), 5301–5309 (2009)
8. Tsai, R., Lenz, R.: Real time versatile robotics hand/eye calibration using 3D machine vision. In: Proceedings of the IEEE International Conference on Robotics and Automation, vol. 1, pp. 554–561 (1988)
9. Hartl, A., Ziegler, S., Navab, N.: Models of detection physics for nuclear probes in freehand SPECT reconstruction. In: Proceedings of IEEE Medical Imaging Conference (IEEE MIC), Knoxville, Tennessee, USA (October 2010)
10. Lasser, T., Ntziachristos, V.: Optimization of 360° projection fluorescence molecular tomography. Medical Image Analysis 11(4), 389–399 (2007)
11. Vogel, J., Reichl, T., Gardiazabal, J., Navab, N., Lasser, T.: Optimization of acquisition geometry for intra-operative tomographic imaging. In: Ayache, N., Delingette, H., Golland, P., Mori, K. (eds.) MICCAI 2012, Part III. LNCS, vol. 7512, pp. 42–49. Springer, Heidelberg (2012)
12. Vetter, C., Lasser, T., Wendler, T., Navab, N.: 1D–3D registration for functional nuclear imaging. In: Fichtinger, G., Martel, A., Peters, T. (eds.) MICCAI 2011, Part I. LNCS, vol. 6891, pp. 227–234. Springer, Heidelberg (2011)
13. Vidal-Sicart, S., Vermeeren, L., Solà, O., Paredes, P., Valdés-Olmos, R.: The use of a portable gamma camera for preoperative lymphatic mapping: a comparison with a conventional gamma camera. Eur. J. Nucl. Med. Mol. Imaging 38(4), 636–641 (2011)
14. Taylor, R., Paul, H., Kazanzides, P., Mittelstadt, B., Hanson, W., Zuhars, J., Williamson, B., Musits, B., Glassman, E., Bargar, W.: Taming the bull: safety in a precise surgical robot. In: Fifth International Conference on Advanced Robotics (ICAR), vol. 1, pp. 865–870 (June 1991)

Robust Real-Time Image-Guided Endoscopy: A New Discriminative Structural Similarity Measure for Video to Volume Registration

Xiongbiao Luo[1], Hirotsugu Takabatake[2], Hiroshi Natori[3], and Kensaku Mori[1]

[1] Information and Communications Headquarters, Nagoya University, Japan
[2] Sapporo Minamisanjo Hospital
[3] Keiwakai Nishioka Hospital, Japan
xiongbiao.luo@gmail.com, kensaku@is.nagoya-u.ac.jp

Abstract. This paper proposes a fully automatic real-time robust image-guided endoscopy method that uses a new discriminative structural similarity measure for pre- and intra-operative registration. Current approaches are limited to clinical applications due to two major bottlenecks: (1) weak continuity, i.e., endoscopic guidance may be blocked since a similarity measure might incorrectly characterize video images and virtual renderings generated from pre-operative volume data, resulting in a registration failure; (2) slow computation, since volume rendering is a time-consuming step in the registration. To address the first drawback, we introduce a robust similarity measure, which uses the degradation of structural information and considers image correlation or structure, luminance, and contrast to characterize images. Moreover, we utilize graphics processing unit techniques to accelerate the volume rendering step. We evaluated our method on patient datasets. The experimental results demonstrated that we provide a promising method, which is possibly applied in the operating room, to accurately and robustly guide endoscopy in real time, particularly the average accuracy of position and orientation was improved from (14.6, 51.2) to (4.45 mm, 12.3°) and the runtime was about 32 frames per second compared to current image-guided methods.

Keywords: Image-Guidance Endoscopy, Endoscope Tracking and Navigation, Video-Volume Registration, Discriminative Structural Similarity.

1 Endoscopic Interventions

Endoscopic interventions are widely performed for cancer diagnosis, e.g., bronchoscopy and endoscopic sinus surgery. Such interventions use endoscopes to insert into the body through natural orifices and observe suspicious regions where biopsies may be performed. However, these interventions in the hands of different skilled endoscopists are the most sensitive procedure for locating tumors since endoscopic video cameras only provide two-dimensional (2-D) image information, which is not enough to determine six-degree-of-freedom (6DoF) position and orientation of an endoscope in a three-dimensional (3-D) space. Moreover, timing of endoscopy depends on physicians' skills; the more time of endoscopy

D. Barratt et al. (Eds.): IPCAI 2013, LNCS 7915, pp. 91–100, 2013.

being operated, the more high risk the patients have. An image-guided endoscopy is promising to address the problems of location and timing of endoscopy.

Image-guided endoscopy registers 2-D video images to 3-D pre-operative data, e.g., computed tomography (CT) or magnetic resonance (MR) images that are usually acquired before interventions, to navigate or locate the endoscope in a reference coordinate system in real time. It usually defines a similarity measure to compute image intensity difference between video and virtual rendering images and runs an optimizer to find the optimal corresponding virtual image [1,2,3]. Compared to commercially available electromagnetically navigated endoscopy [4,5], it has several interesting advantages including cost-efficient, without additional setups, little influence from respiratory motion, and without inherent system or dynamic errors. Unfortunately, two main weaknesses limit image-guided endoscopy to apply in operation rooms: (1) guidance discontinuity and (2) large amount of calculation. The former is caused by problematic endoscopic images (e.g., local luminance and contrast changes) that may easily collapse the registration since the similarity measure may not adapt itself to these changes. The latter results from volume rendering to generate virtual images, blocking a real-time guidance procedure where at lest 30 frames are processed in a second. Even though many papers have been published in the literature [1,3], more accurate and effective methods to tackle these weaknesses are still expected for the robust real-time image-guided endoscopy.

This work realized a robust real-time image-guided endoscopy. To accurately register 2-D video images and 3-D CT volume, we proposed a new discriminative structural similarity (DSSIM) measure. The similarity function is a key element that is expected to precisely characterize intensity difference under a dynamic environment. DSSIM can adapt itself successfully to image changes due to non-linear illumination, specular- or inter-reflection, or collision with the organ walls in endoscopy. Moreover, since generating 2-D virtual images is time-consuming, we use graphics processing unit (GPU) techniques to accelerate our method up to 32 frames per second (fps), which meets the real-time requirement ($\geq$ 30 fps).

Several highlights of this work are summarized as follows. First, we modified a measure of structural similarity (SSIM) to DSSIM that is robust and accurate for a video-volume registration. We extended a new application of SSIM in computer assisted interventions. Furthermore, to best of our knowledge, no methods were published as real-time image-guided endoscopy using image registration methods before. We reported a fully automatic image-guided endoscopy in real time. Additionally, our method is suitable to other endoscopies (e.g., conchoscope).

2   Proposed Approaches

Our proposed approach to guide endoscopic interventions and determine endoscope 6DoF location information comprises of several main steps: (1) automatically initializing the guided procedure, (2) formulating the discriminative structural similarity measure, and (3) performing video-volume registration for continuous endoscope guidance. Fig. 1 shows the flowchart of our proposed method.

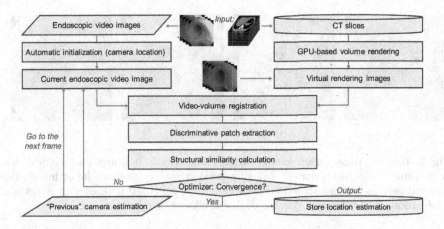

Fig. 1. The processing flowchart of our proposed method for endoscope guidance

2.1 Automatic Initialization

Endoscopic guidance must be initialized before continuous navigation. It is hard to perform a manual initialization that takes much time during examination. It is also somewhat difficult to use fiducials to align from patient to CT spaces. For surgical requirements, we here introduce a fully automatic initialization method on the basis of airway tree structures and manifold learning.

First, we segment CT images to obtain the centerlines of the trachea, the left main bronchus, and the right main bronchus with their start and end positions, $(\mathbf{s}_t, \mathbf{e}_t)$, $(\mathbf{s}_l, \mathbf{e}_l)$, and $(\mathbf{s}_r, \mathbf{e}_r)$, before an endoscopic intervention. The carina position should be either $\mathbf{e}_t$ or $\mathbf{s}_l$ or $\mathbf{s}_r$.

Next, we generate a set of virtual images by updating position $\mathbf{p}_i$ and orientation $\mathbf{o}_i(\mathbf{o}_i^x, \mathbf{o}_i^y, \mathbf{o}_i^z)$ of a virtual camera in the CT space ($\alpha \in [0.5\ 0.9]$):

$$\mathbf{p}_i = \mathbf{s}_t + \frac{\alpha(\mathbf{e}_t - \mathbf{s}_t)}{\|\mathbf{e}_t - \mathbf{s}_t\|}, \ \mathbf{o}_i^z = \frac{(\mathbf{e}_t - \mathbf{s}_t)}{\|\mathbf{e}_t - \mathbf{s}_t\|}, \ \mathbf{o}_i^y = \frac{(\mathbf{e}_l - \mathbf{s}_l)}{\|\mathbf{e}_l - \mathbf{s}_l\|} \times \frac{(\mathbf{e}_r - \mathbf{s}_r)}{\|\mathbf{e}_r - \mathbf{s}_r\|}, \quad (1)$$

where, $\mathbf{o}_i^x = \mathbf{o}_i^z \times \mathbf{o}_i^y, \mathbf{o}_i^y$, and $\mathbf{o}_i^z$ are the direction vectors of the virtual camera.

Finally, we use a manifold learning method to construct the subspace for those generated virtual images with different camera poses (position and orientation parameters) [6]. During the intervention, the physician can initially locate the endoscope around the carina of the airways and embedded the current video image to the subspace·and find the optimal initialization to start a navigation.

2.2 Discriminative Structural Similarity

The similarity measure is a core of image registration. It is supposed to accurately and robustly represent image changes (distortion), e.g., illumination and motion blurring. We propose a discriminative structural similarity measure that

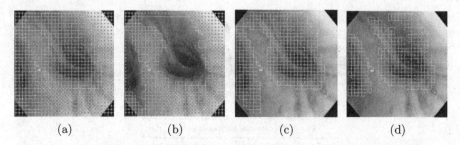

(a)   (b)   (c)   (d)

Fig. 2. Discriminative region extraction (a *yellow square* indicates one patch and a *green point* is one patch center): (a) all separated patches from an input image, (b) removed patches without structural information, (c) remained patches with structural information, (d) finally used patches during similarity computation.

takes incomplete correlation, luminance and contrast distortion into consideration to model image changes. *Discriminative* here means specific structures such as bifurcations and folds inside the airways. Since the structural information is very useful for the similarity calculation, we first extract discriminative regions.

Discriminative Region Extraction. For an image with $W \times H$ pixels, we divide it into $U \times V$ patches. One patch $P_{u,v}$ with $\frac{W}{U} \times \frac{H}{V}$ pixels is presented by:

$$P_{u,v} = \{(c_x, c_y), u \in U, v \in V\}, \tag{2}$$

where c_x and c_y are the patch center coordinates. We define two variables: intensity variance $\sigma_{u,v}$ and contrast $\omega_{u,v}$ that indicates the tone of the highlights and lighter areas, to check whether $P_{u,v}$ includes the structural information:

$$\sigma_{u,v}^2 = \frac{1}{|P_{u,v}|} \sum_{P_{u,v}} \left(P_{u,v}(x,y) - \bar{P}_{u,v} \right)^2, \; \omega_{u,v} = \frac{1}{|P_{u,v}|} \sum_{P_{u,v}} \Psi \left(P_{u,v}(x,y) \right), \tag{3}$$

where (x,y), $|P_{u,v}|$, and $\bar{P}_{u,v}$ denote one pixel coordinates, the pixel number, and the average intensity in patch $P_{u,v}$, respectively. Function $\Psi \left(P_{u,v}(x,y) \right)$, which depends on the pixel color information of saturation $S(x,y)$ and lightness $L(x,y)$ in the hue-saturation-lightness (HSL) color model, is defined to evaluate whether pixel (x,y) belongs to the highlights and lighter areas or not:

$$\Psi \left(P_{u,v}(x,y) \right) = \begin{cases} 1 & S(x,y) \leq \beta_S \; and \; L(x,y) \geq \delta_L \\ 0 & otherwise \end{cases}, \tag{4}$$

where β_S and δ_L are two pre-determined thresholds. We remove the white patches without structural information by $\omega_{u,v} \geq \epsilon_\omega$ (a fixed constant), descendingly sort the remained patches in terms of $\sigma_{u,v}$, and choose $\lambda \cdot U \cdot V$ patches for the similarity calculation. Fig. 2 shows the discriminative patch detection.

Structural Similarity Function. A similarity function seeks to correctly depict pixel difference between distorted and reference images in the registration. Image distortion usually results from structure (correlation), luminance, and contrast changes. Based on the work of SSIM [7], we introduce the similarity function M into the volume-video registration for guided interventions as:

$$M = \underbrace{\frac{\sigma_{d,r} + C_1}{\sigma_d \sigma_r + C_1}}_{Structure} \cdot \underbrace{\frac{2\xi_d \xi_r + C_2}{\xi_d^2 + \xi_r^2 + C_2}}_{Luminance} \cdot \underbrace{\frac{2\sigma_d \sigma_r + C_3}{\sigma_d^2 + \sigma_r^2 + C_3}}_{Contrast}, \tag{5}$$

where $\sigma_{d,r}$ is the correlation between distorted and reference images; ξ_d and ξ_r are the intensity mean; σ_d and σ_r are the intensity variance, respectively (constants: C_1, C_2, and C_3). Three elements in Eq. 5 were demonstrated to successfully characterize image changes [7]. By $C_3 = 2C_1$, we rewrote Eq. 5 as:

$$M = \frac{(2\sigma_{d,r} + C_1)(2\xi_d \xi_r + C_2)}{(\sigma_d^2 + \sigma_r^2 + C_1)(\xi_d^2 + \xi_r^2 + C_2)}. \tag{6}$$

After choosing $\lambda \cdot U \cdot V$ discriminative regions, similarity $DSSIM(I_k, I_{CT})$ between k-th video sequence I_k and CT-based virtual image I_{CT} is computed by:

$$DSSIM(I_k, I_{CT}) = \frac{1}{\lambda \cdot U \cdot V} \sum_{P_{u,v} \in \lambda \cdot U \cdot V} \frac{1}{|P_{u,v}|} \sum_{P_{u,v}} \hat{M}_{u,v}, \tag{7}$$

$$\hat{M}_{u,v} = \frac{\left(2\sigma_{k,CT}^{u,v} + C_1\right)(2\xi_k^{u,v} \xi_{CT}^{u,v} + C_2)}{((\sigma_k^{u,v})^2 + (\sigma_{CT}^{u,v})^2 + C_1)((\xi_k^{u,v})^2 + (\xi_{CT}^{u,v})^2 + C_2)}. \tag{8}$$

The DSSIM measure will be demonstrated to very robust and accurate for registering video and CT-based virtual images from our experimental results.

Remarks on the DSSIM Measure. Image structural or discriminative information is very useful for the similarity calculation since it describes the pixel dependency that involves significant information about visual structures. Hence, a robust similarity measure should be able to characterize visual structural information in images. Moreover, image similarity should be computed locally but not globally, i.e., an image should be divided into many patches and the similarity of each patch is calculated and added up to the finial similarity. The similarity's locality is better than its globality since it yields several practical situations, e.g., dynamic of image statistical features, image distortion being independent or dependent of local characteristics, the human vision system being sensitive to local structures, and a variable image quality map related to local quality measurement. Additionally, a good measure should be insensitive to luminance and contrast changes. DSSIM can meet three requirements of a good similarity measure: (1) usage of structural information (2) locality, and (3) adaptation of luminance or contrast distortion. We extract discriminative structures (bifurcations or folds) in local regions and compute the local similarity of the patches whose luminance or contrast distortion was modeled.

2.3   Video-Volume Registration

For a continuous endoscopic navigation, we must perform the video-volume registration (V^2R) to determine the spatial transformation between the video and

CT volume coordinate systems during the image-guided endoscopic intervention. Such a spatial transformation involves with the 6DoF parameters of position and orientation of the endoscope located somewhere in the airways.

Suppose that $^{CT}\mathbf{T}_V^k$ with position $^{CT}\mathbf{t}_V$ and rotation matrix $^{CT}\mathbf{R}_V$ is the transformation matrix from video to volume at frame k. To estimate $^{CT}\mathbf{T}_V^{k+1}$, we formulate V^{2}R as an optimization process on the basis of the proposed DSSIM measure and determine the changeable transformation parameter $\Delta^{CT}\mathbf{T}_V^{k+1}$ by:

$$\Delta^{CT}\mathbf{T}_V^{k+1} = \arg\,max_{\Delta^{CT}\mathbf{T}_V^{k+1}} DSSIM\left(I_k, I_{CT}(^{CT}\mathbf{T}_V^k \cdot \Delta^{CT}\mathbf{T}_V^{k+1})\right), \quad (9)$$

where virtual image $I_{CT}(\cdot)$ is generated on the basis of virtual camera parameters $^{CT}\mathbf{T}_V^k \cdot \Delta^{CT}\mathbf{T}_V^{k+1}$. By running an optimizer, we find optimal $\Delta^{CT}\check{\mathbf{T}}_V^{k+1}$ to maximize the similarity between images I_{k+1} and $I_{CT}(^{CT}\mathbf{T}_V^k \cdot \Delta^{CT}\check{\mathbf{T}}_V^{k+1})$.

Note that the initialization of $\Delta^{CT}\mathbf{T}_V^{k+1}$ is important to the optimizer, as discussed in [3]. It can be initialized as an identity matrix. Such an initialization will lose the temporal coherence between two consecutive video frames, possibly resulting in a guidance failure. Video image textures or features can be used to compensate such losing. However, such a compensation takes much time. In this work, we determine the initialization empirically. We clarify that typical translating and rotating speeds of an endoscope is 10.0 mm and 20 degrees per second. An endoscopic camera is usually at frame rate of 30 fps. Therefore, interframe speeds τ and ϕ of translation and rotation are about 0.33 mm and 0.66 degrees per frame ($\tau = 0.33$ mm and $\phi = 0.66$ degrees). Hence, we can initialize $\Delta^{CT}\mathbf{T}_V^{k+1}$ by the following equations:

$$\Delta^{CT}\mathbf{T}_V^{k+1} = \begin{pmatrix} \Delta^{CT}\mathbf{R}_V^{k+1} & \Delta^{CT}\mathbf{t}_V^{k+1} \\ \mathbf{0}^T & 1 \end{pmatrix}_{4\times 4}, \quad (10)$$

$$\Delta^{CT}\mathbf{t}_V^{k+1} = [\tau\ \tau\ \tau]^T, \quad \Delta^{CT}\mathbf{R}_V^{k+1} = \begin{pmatrix} b^2 & a^2 b - ab & ab^2 + a^2 \\ ab & a^3 + b^2 & a^2 b - ab \\ -a & ab & b^2 \end{pmatrix}_{3\times 3}, \quad (11)$$

where the variables of matrix $\Delta^{CT}\mathbf{R}_V^{k+1}$ are defined as: $a = \sin\phi$ and $b = \cos\phi$.

3   Experimental Settings

We validated our proposed method on six cases of patient datasets: (1) endoscopic video images, whose sizes were 360×370 and 256×263 pixels, were recorded at a frame rate of 30 fps, and (2) CT volumes were acquired by space parameters of 512×512 pixels, 72-351 slices, 2.0-5.0-mm slice thickness.

We implemented our method on a Dell Precision Workstation that was equipped with Intel (R) Xeon(R) CPU X5355 2.66 GHz × 8, NVIDIA GeForce 8800 GTX, and 16.0 GB memory and installed with the Windows 7 64-bit operating system and the NVIDIA CUDA 4.2 toolkit. We investigate two image-based

Table 1. Quantitative results of the guidance accuracy of the two methods in terms of position and orientation errors between the estimates and ground truth

Patient data (Frames)	Comparison of (position, orientation) of the two methods	
	MoMSE	DSSIM
Case A (379)	(31.2±25.8 mm, 38.8±29.3°)	(9.08±6.88 mm, 12.4±8.00°)
Case B (1000)	(12.4±7.84 mm, 72.8±52.3°)	(2.88±1.62 mm, 10.8±6.53°)
Case C (449)	(4.75±2.99 mm, 10.0±5.80°)	(4.35±2.77 mm, 9.29±4.50°)
Case D (2650)	(10.4±5.70 mm, 66.6±35.4°)	(2.32±1.81 mm, 8.67±7.21°)
Case E (450)	(13.8±11.7 mm, 23.9±18.6°)	(4.64±2.75 mm, 17.7±14.7°)
Case F (2000)	(15.3±14.3 mm, 45.6±28.5°)	(3.42±3.07 mm, 14.2±12.3°)
Average	**(14.6±11.4 mm, 51.2±28.3°)**	**(4.45±3.15 mm, 12.3±8.88°)**

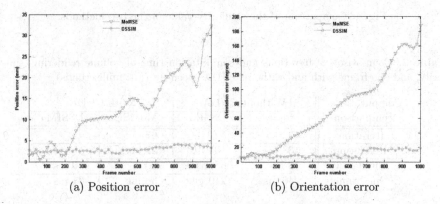

(a) Position error   (b) Orientation error

Fig. 3. Navigation position and orientation errors of the two methods on Case B was plotted against ground truth by every 20 frames

methods: (1) MoMSE: a method using a modified mean square error similarity measure [1], (2) DSSIM: our method, as discussed in Section 2. To evaluate the guidance accuracy, we generate ground truth data by manually adjusting the position and orientation of the virtual camera to qualitatively align video and CT-driven virtual images. Additionally, we set parameters: $U = V = 30$, $\lambda = 0.3$, $\beta_S = 0.6$, $\delta_L = 0.7$, and $\epsilon_\omega = 0.9$ during discriminative region extraction.

4   Results

Table 1 lists the guidance accuracy by computing the position and orientation errors between ground truth and the estimates. The mean position and orientation errors of our approach were 4.45 mm and 12.3°, which are significantly better than 14.6 mm and 51.2° of the MoMSE-based method. Fig. 3 plots the guidance accuracy of the MoMSE- and DSSIM-based methods on Case B. Fig. 5 shows some video images of Case D and their corresponding virtual images generated from the estimated results. Fig. 4 compares the similarity between video and virtual images, demonstrating that the visualization quality of the DSSIM-based method is absolutely better than the MoMSE-based method (Fig. 5).

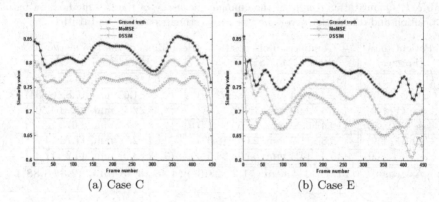

(a) Case C   (b) Case E

Fig. 4. Comparison of the similarity value of the two methods.

Table 2. Comparison of iterations and computation time of volume rendering, similarity, and one frame with and without CUDA speed-up (ms: milliseconds)

Computation comparison	Without CUDA		With CUDA	
	MoMSE	DSSIM	MoMSE	DSSIM
Iterations	77	52	67	49
Rendering	138 ms	104 ms	22 ms	15 ms
Similarity	38 ms	68 ms	6 ms	10 ms
One frame	246 ms	219 ms	38 ms	31 ms

4351   4576   4801   5026   05251   5476   5701   5926   6151   6376   6601   6825

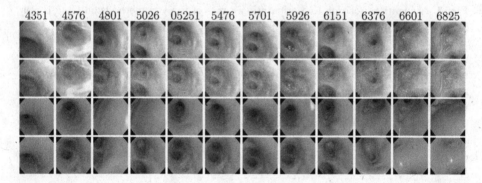

Fig. 5. Visual comparison of guidance results of Case D. Top row shows uniformly selected frame numbers, and second row shows their corresponding video images. Third row gives the results of discriminative region extraction. Fourth and fifth rows display virtual images based on the estimates from the MoMSE- and DSSIM-based methods, respectively. Our method shows better performance.

More interestingly, our approach can be implemented in real time using GPU techniques. After accelerating by GPU, the DSSIM-based approach needs about 31 milliseconds per frame (mpf), i.e., processing about 32 fps, which exceeds the

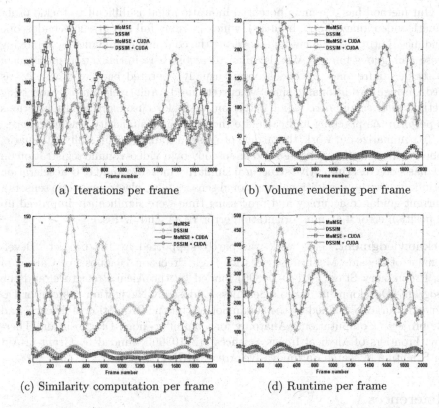

(a) Iterations per frame   (b) Volume rendering per frame

(c) Similarity computation per frame   (d) Runtime per frame

Fig. 6. Comparison of the computational times of the two methods on Case F

clinical requirement of 30 fps. The MoMSE-based method can process about 26 fps (38 mpf), slightly being lower than the real-time need (Table 2 and Fig. 6).

5 Discussion and Conclusion

We realized a real-time endoscope guidance with a more robust and accurate navigation. We believe that the effectiveness lies in the DSSIM's robustness. Sine the visualization quality of guidance results (i.e., virtual images generated from endoscope location parameters) depends on the human visual system (HVS) that is very sensitive to structural information in images, a good similarity measure should approximate structural information changes as accurate as possible. MoMSE computes pixel difference to approximate image distortion but hardly fits to HVS. DSSIM, which use structural information changes to characterize image distortion, follows HVS well. Moreover, DSSIM can adapt itself to luminance and contrast dynamics, as proved in our experimental results. Additionally, the runtime, which was improved to the real-time level, is mainly attributed to GPU techniques. We believe that the similarity measure that makes convergence fast can also reduce the runtime (Fig. 6). Even though DSSIM is computed by more time than MoMSE, its robustness makes iterations reduced in optimization.

Our method has one main potential limitation that is difficult to tackle problematic video images (e.g., bubbles), which possibly fail a continuous endoscope guidance. Future work includes recovering the continuous guidance by removing these ambiguous images. We also plan to revoke a re-initialization mechanism to tackle failure since an endoscope is usually operated back to where it has flied through. Additionally, since we current used a relatively simple processing method in discriminative region detection, we seek to use more robust functions to perform the patching and calculate the inter-pixel similarity among images.

To summarize our work, this article proposes a framework of a fully automatic, robust, and real-time image-guided endoscopy by a video-volume registration on the basis of a discriminative structural similarity measure and GPU acceleration techniques, without additional positional sensors (e.g., electromagnetic sensors). Current guidance accuracy and processing time were significantly improved up to position error 4.45 mm, orientation error 12.3°, and 32 fps.

Acknowledgment. This work was partly supported by the project "Development of Bedside Medical Devices for High Precision Diagnosis of Cancer in Its Preliminary Stage" (01-D-D0806) funded by the Aichi Prefecture, and the program "Development of Scale Seamless Endoscopy Navigation System for Diagnostic Surgery" funded by the Japan Society for the Promotion of Science, and the project "Computational Anatomy for Computer-aided Diagnosis and Therapy: Frontiers of Medical Image Sciences" (21103006) funded by Grant-in-Aid for Scientific Research on Innovative Areas, MEXT, Japan.

References

1. Deguchi, D., et al.: Selective image similarity measure for bronchoscope tracking based on image registration. MedIA 13(4), 621–633 (2009)
2. Mirota, D.J., et al.: A system for video-based navigation for endoscopic endonasal skull base surgery. IEEE TMI 31(4), 963–976 (2012)
3. Luo, X., et al.: Development and comparison of new hybrid motion tracking for bronchoscopic navigation. MedIA 16(3), 577–596 (2012)
4. Schwarz, Y., et al.: Real-time electromagnetic navigation bronchoscopy to peripheral lung lesions using overlaid CT images: The first human study. Chest 129(4), 988–994
5. Luó, X., Reichl, T., Feuerstein, M., Kitasaka, T., Mori, K.: Modified hybrid bronchoscope tracking based on sequential Monte Carlo sampler: dynamic phantom validation. In: Kimmel, R., Klette, R., Sugimoto, A. (eds.) ACCV 2010, Part III. LNCS, vol. 6494, pp. 409–421. Springer, Heidelberg (2011)
6. Luo, X., Kitasaka, T., Mori, K.: ManiSMC: A new method using manifold modeling and sequential Monte Carlo sampler for boosting navigated bronchoscopy. In: Fichtinger, G., Martel, A., Peters, T. (eds.) MICCAI 2011, Part III. LNCS, vol. 6893, pp. 248–255. Springer, Heidelberg (2011)
7. Wang, Z., et al.: Image quality assessment: From error visibility to structural similarity. IEEE TIP 13(4), 600–612 (2004)

Declustering n-Connected Components for Segmentation of Iodine Implants in C-Arm Fluoroscopy Images

Chiara Amat di San Filippo[5], Gabor Fichtinger[1], William James Morris[2],
Septimiu E. Salcudean[3], Ehsan Dehghan[4], and Pascal Fallavollita[5]

[1] Queen's University, Kingston, Canada
[2] Vancouver Cancer Center, Vancouver, Canada
[3] University of British Columbia, Vancouver, Canada
[4] Philips Healthcare, New York, USA
[5] Technische Universität München, Germany
{Filippo,fallavol}@in.tum.de, gabor@cs.queensu.ca,
jmorris@bccancer.bc.ca, tims@ece.ubc.ca,
ehsan.dehghan@philips.com

Abstract. Dynamic dosimetry is becoming the standard to evaluate the quality of radioactive implants during brachytherapy. It is essential to obtain a 3D visualization of the implanted seeds and their relative position to the prostate. For this, a robust and precise segmentation of the seeds in 2D X-ray is required. First, implanted seeds are segmented using a region-based implicit active contour approach. Then, n-seed clusters are resolved using an efficient template based approach. A collection of 55 C-arm images from 10 patients are used to validate the proposed algorithm. Compared to manual ground-truth segmentation of 6002 seeds, 98.7% of seeds were automatically detected and declustered showing a false-positive rate of only 1.7%. Results indicate the proposed method is able to perform the identification and annotation processes of seeds on par with a human expert, constituting a viable alternative to the traditional manual segmentation approach.

1 Introduction

With an estimated 240,890 new cases in 2011, prostate cancer is the most common cancer among men in the United States, accounting for 29% of their cancers [1]. Brachytherapy, a definitive treatment for early stage prostate cancer, demonstrates excellent long-term disease-free survival and is chosen by over 60, 000 men annually. The brachytherapy procedure entails permanent implantation of small radioactive seeds, such as ^{125}I, ^{103}Pd, or ^{137}Cs, into the prostate to eliminate the cancer via radiation. Before the operation, the seed positions are planned using a transrectal ultrasound (TRUS) volume. The goal of the planning is to cover the target gland with a prescribed dose of radiation, while sparing the healthy surrounding tissue such as urethra and rectum. In current brachytherapy interventions, seed placement is performed under visual guidance from TRUS and further assessed with the acquisitions of multiple C-arm fluoroscopy images. Intraoperative dynamic dosimetry, the fusion of both TRUS and fluoroscopy data, would enable physicians to account for deviations from

D. Barratt et al. (Eds.): IPCAI 2013, LNCS 7915, pp. 101–110, 2013.
© Springer-Verlag Berlin Heidelberg 2013

the initial seeds placement plan and tailor the remaining dose so as to eradicate the cancer while minimizing harm to the surrounding healthy tissues [2].

1.1   Intra-operative Dynamic Dosimetry Workflow

The following workflow closely reflects intraoperative dosimetry analysis and optimization (see Figure 1). The oncologist will acquire a number of transrectal ultrasound images until they feel it is time to verify implant position and dosimetric values. At that point, the acquired slices are compounded into a 3D volume. A C-arm fluoroscopy device is moved near the patient table and several X-ray images are acquired showing implant position. The C-arm images are pre-processed and the precise seed segmentations can be calculated using segmentation techniques. Next, seed correspondence between the acquired C-arm images is performed and subsequent 3D reconstruction of the seeds is realized as in [11]. The 3D ultrasound volume is then registered to the 3D seed reconstruction using a state-of-the art method as in [12, 13]. The oncologist can visually assess the multimodal fused data and determine whether there are under-dosed regions (cold spots) or regions with high risk of over-radiation. Lastly, dynamic dosimetry is inherently executed since the oncologist could change the planned position of the remaining seeds and add new seeds if required. To achieve suitable dynamic dosimetry intraoperatively precise seed segmentation must be achieved. Unfortunately, modern C-arm images are still afflicted with low signal-to-noise ratios and are characterized by illumination inhomogeneity [3]. Using thresholding algorithms would yield poor results [4]. Lastly, since many implants overlap— as many as five seed clusters in some scenarios— techniques to resolve these clusters into their constituent components need further investigation.

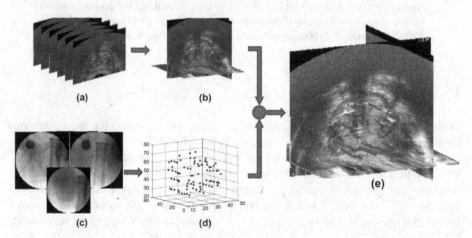

Fig. 1. Dynamic dosimetry outline. (a): Several ultrasound images of the prostate. (b): 3D ultrasound volume. (c): C-arm images showing seeds. (d): Seeds reconstructed in 3D. (e): Registered seeds overlaid on the US volume. Seeds are shown as red capsules Image taken from the authors in [12].

1.2 Existing Segmentation Algorithms of Implants

Brachytherapy seed segmentation in C-arm fluoroscopy images is a well-known topic in research practice [3-6]. For brevity, we summarize some of the key contributors in this topic. In Lam *et al.* [3], it is possible to observe the usage of a spoke transform to facilitate seed segmentation. In Tubic *et al.* [4], the morphological top-hat transform was used to normalize image illumination, in order to prepare the image for thresholding which was achieved through the bidimensional entropy method. Grouped pixels, thus potential seeds clusters, were identified using area, width, and length statistics of the clusters and subsequently declustered using a simulated annealing type algorithm. In Kuo *et al.* [5], a top-hat by reconstruction algorithm followed by thresholding via Otsu's method was employed. Overlapping seeds were identified- but not separated- by calculating the sum of the intensities of each pixel group and comparing it to the median sum. In the most recent state-of-the-art method, Moult *et al.* [6] used top-hat, Gaussian and Kirsch filters in combination. Afterwards, they used an implicit active contour algorithm to produce an image showing only the seeds. Finally, a declustering algorithm to decompose only two-seed clusters was introduced via a template-based scheme. All of the above works suffer from distinct limitations: (i) in [5] the authors consider only palladium seed segmentation, (ii) in all algorithmic steps require manual intervention for image cropping and definition of algorithm parameter thresholds and (iii) only $n=2$ seed clusters were accounted for which significantly reduces accuracy of seed reconstruction.

1.3 Contributions

According to Radiotherapy in Practice Brachytherapy: *"[t]he most frequently used isotope for permanent seed implantation in brachytherapy is iodine-125* [10]." Different implants require different segmentation schemes due to their shape and size— thus ^{103}Pd, or ^{137}Cs segmentation algorithms cannot be applied to iodine seeds which are longer in size. Consequently, the existing two-cluster solutions cannot be reduced for general clinical practice. It is clinically unacceptable to perform manual segmentation on the seeds, intra-operatively during the procedure, for every C-arm image of an implant (i.e. almost 5 seeds/C-arm image in [6]). This results in long procedure times and invites human operator errors. Clinical experience proves that n-cluster seed segmentation is required for a viable clinical implementation of intra-operative implant reconstruction and dosimetry. In this paper, a template matching technique that allows for fast and accurate n-seed cluster decomposition is proposed.

2 Implicit Active Contours and Initial Preprocessing

To segment the iodine brachytherapy implants, a region-based implicit active contour model by Li *et al.* [7] is used. Generally medical images have intensity inhomogeneity; hence the model proposed by Li *et al.* is suitable as it accounts for variances in image illumination and additionally eliminates the re-initialization process making this algorithm automatic. The initial segmentation can be summarized by the following four steps:

STEP 1: the X-ray image is filtered producing a processed image on which the active contour will be evolved. In this step, a morphological top-hat filter with rectangular structuring element is applied. The structuring element has dimension 12×2 pixels with longer y-axis length. We made the fitting assumption that implanted seeds in X-ray are rectangular in shape and closer to an upright orientation. It is impossible to insert and deposit a seed horizontally when guiding needle insertion using the needle template during brachytherapy.

STEP 2: the image that is used to initialize the active contour is generated here thereby eliminating the need for a manually defined ROI. This initialization image is formed using a top-hat filter, blurring the original X-ray with a Gaussian filter and employing a Kirsch edge filter [8]. For all trials the Kirsch filter threshold was $t_0 = 5$. Once the binarized edge image is formed, black-white (BW), the initial level set function ϕ^0 is defined as:

$$\phi^0(i,j) = \begin{cases} -c_0 & \text{if} \quad BW(i,j) = 1 \\ \\ c_0 & \text{elsewhere} \end{cases} \tag{1}$$

where $c_0 = 2$ as indicated in [7].

STEP 3: evolves the level set function for 70 iterations, after which a resulting binary image is obtained containing the seeds and possibly some lingering noise. For all trials, the energy functional parameters were set as those defined by the author in [7].

STEP 4: eliminates any remaining noise in the image. Connected regions < 20 pixels are discarded since their areas are below the assumed area of an implanted seed. Also, if the region width is larger than the region length, we discard as well, since implants are always closer to an upright position. Mean statistics are subsequently calculated similar to the state-of-the art method of [6]. Mean pixel area is determined by the number of pixels contained in all clusters. This value is divided by the number of connected components in the X-ray image. Lastly, regions of the image that deviate significantly from the mean statistics are removed. The statistics were formulated by analyzing the mean pixel area (MPA) of seed groups within X-ray images. The pixel groupings in this paper were set to [0.5, 5] times MPA. A value of five suggests at most 5 seed clusters whereas a value of ½ suggests the lower limit possibility of a region being a seed. This resulting image is used when applying the declustering algorithm described in the following section.

3   Declustering n-Connected Components

In the image, it is expected to find certain pixels that define two or more seed clusters. This fact motivates the introduction of seed declustering techniques to resolve such groupings. First, we briefly describe a method to reduce the search space as proposed in [4, 6]. Second, we outline the steps involved in discerning the *n*-seed clusters based on area and length measures. Lastly, a general *n*-seed declustering scheme is outlined.

3.1   Search Space Reduction and Cluster-Discerning Criteria

In order to make the declustering algorithm faster, a technique to reduce the search space within the C-arm images is introduced. The declustering technique is based on matching a set of template seeds to the overlapping seed group of interest [4]. The problem of this method is prohibitively large search space, hence to overcome this limitation, translation of the model template is not allowed and instead a set of 3 anchor points uniformly spaced in the shortest side of the pixel group is considered. This produces a search space reduced by over 99.96% [6]. In this paper, the clusters are identified and discriminated based on the area and length statistics of the clusters. We calculated the mean pixel area **A** (i.e. the area that a single seed should approximately have), calculated the mean pixel length **L** (i.e. the length that a single seed should approximately have and equal to the major axis length of the minimal enclosed bounding ellipse of the connected region). Then, we carefully selected the parameters $n_1 < n_2 < n_3 < n_4 < n_5 \in R$ and $m_1 < m_2 < m_3 < m_4 < m_5 \in R$ such that

- [(if $A \geq n_1 \cdot A$) and ($A < n_2 \cdot A$)] *or* [($l \geq m_1 \cdot l$) and ($l < m_2 \cdot l$)] – *two seed cluster*
- [(if $A \geq n_2 \cdot A$) and ($A < n_3 \cdot A$)] *or* [($l \geq m_2 \cdot l$) and ($l < m_3 \cdot l$)] – *three seed cluster*

The same reasoning is used to discern clusters of four and five seeds. In the implemented procedure the choice of values was determined empirically by analyzing a subset of C-arm images: $n_1=m_1=$ 1.3; $n_2= m_2=$ 1.9; $n_3=m_3=$ 3.1; $n_4=m_4=$ 4.0; $n_5=m_5=4.5$. Through these values all possible cluster shapes can be accounted for (i.e. Y-shape, etc.). We randomly selected a subset of 5 images to train and arrive at the above values. A visual inspection of the subset of images revealed seed projections having 'close enough' geometric similarities capturing population variability.

Template Seeds for matching: A template seeds are a rectangle of size 5 × 22 pixels (i.e. 1.0 x 4.4 mm using a pixel spacing equal to 0.2013mm) determined empirically by visualizing a sub-sample of projected seeds in the C-arm images. To achieve improved precision not just one template fixation point is used, but three, lying on the shortest side of the seed. A set of possible rotations $R = \{k \cdot (\pi/16) \rightarrow k \in 0, \ldots, 15\}$ is also considered and the templates which have the highest intersection with the pixel cluster is selected as the matching one.

3.2   *n*-Seed Declustering Framework

The graphical outline of the procedure can be seen in Figures 2-3. The pixels of the *n*-seed cluster are labelled with the number **c**. The pixels p_1^* and p_n^* are defined as the most distant ones in the cluster (Figure 2a). Using the two-seed declustering algorithm in [6], the pixels p_1^* and p_n^* belong respectively to two different seeds clusters s_1

and s_n. The pixels belonging clusters s_1 and s_n are detected (Figure 2b) and only the ones belonging to s_n and relabelled with the number $c + 1$. The remaining pixels belonging to the original cluster stay untouched and the cluster is now composed of $(n - 1)$ seeds (Figure 3a). Before starting the next iteration just the connected component of the cluster is selected, (see Figure 4). The two-seed declustering algorithm is applied on the connected component of the cluster, and the pixels p_1^* and p_{n-1}^* belong respectively to two different seeds of the cluster s_1 and s_{n-1}.

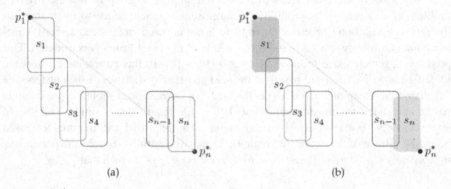

(a)   (b)

Fig. 2. (a) Cluster of n seeds, the points p_1^* and p_n^* are the most distant in the cluster, they belong respectively to seed s_1 and s_n. (b) Seeds s_1 and s_n are detected

The pixels belonging to s_{n-1} are detected and relabelled with the number $c + 2$. At step k, seed s_1 and s_{n-k+1} will be detected with the two-seed declustering algorithm, and only s_{n-k+1} is relabelled with number $c + k$. This procedure is repeated $n - 1$ times. In the last step $k = n - 1$, the most distant pixels p_1^* and p_2^* belong respectively to the last two seeds of the cluster s_1 and s_2 (see Figure 3b). Consequently, the two-seed declustering can be used and the original n-seed cluster has been successfully declustered.

We observe that seed s_1 has been detected $n - 1$ times using template matching and this is an unwanted side-effect of the algorithm and leaves open space for further improvements. In this paper, this problem does not affect the computational cost as we consider only cases in which $n \leq 5$. An improved version of the generalized n-seed declustering algorithm follows. In every iteration k of the algorithm, the pixels belonging to seeds s_1 and s_{n-k+1} are relabeled with numbers $c + 2k - 1$ and $c + 2k$.

In each step, 2 seeds are extracted from the cluster enabling only $\left\lceil \frac{n-1}{2} \right\rceil$ iterations. The last step will be different for the case of n being an even or odd number: if n is odd, there is only one remaining seed labeled with $c \rightarrow$ end algorithm; n is even signifying there are two seeds remaining labeled with $c \rightarrow$ apply the two-seed algorithm. For brevity, the workflow of a three-seed declustering framework is presented in Figure 4 and shown iteratively using a preprocessed clinical scenario.

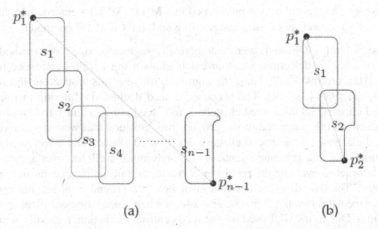

(a)   (b)

Fig. 3. (a) Seed s_n is relabeled and the cluster is formed only from seeds s_1 to s_{n-1}. The most distant points in the cluster are now p_1^* and p_{n-1}^*. (b) The procedure is applied until only two seeds remain at which point [6] is applied.

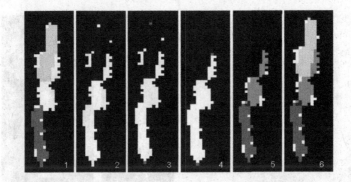

Fig. 4. Declustering workflow for a three-seed grouping. (1) A three-seed cluster where the two most distant seeds are detected using a two-seed clustering technique. (2) One of the seeds is relabeled (i.e. it does not belong to the cluster anymore). (3) The most distant points u* and v* are wrongly selected. (4) The most distant points u* and q* are now correctly selected considering just the connected component of the pixel cluster. (5) The two-seed algorithm is applied again. (6) The three-seed declustering is now complete.

4   Evaluation and Results

Datasets: We validated the proposed segmentation and declustering method on 55 clinical images from 10 patients. One observer segmented the iodine seeds in the clinical images. As per all manual segmentation tasks, the general rule was to select the center point of a seed to the best of their ability. A total of 6002 seed centroids were manually segmented and these are considered the ground-truth seed coordinates for comparison.

Processing: The algorithm was prototyped in a MATLAB/C++ environment having a runtime of 50 seconds per C-arm image using an Intel®Core™ i7 computer.

Results: In total, 5918 seeds were automatically segmented using our method which results in a 98.7% detection rate. Our calculations using a 95% confidence interval, with $p < 0.05$, returns 0.448. Thus, the high and low intervals around our mean detection rate are [98.14, 99.04]. The proposed n-seed declustering algorithm found 554 two-seed clusters, 68 three-seed clusters, 2 four-seed clusters and 1 five-seed cluster. These results were compared to the ground truth clusters, that were respectively 511 two-seed clusters, 56 three-seed clusters, 3 four-seed clusters and 0 five-seed cluster, confirming that the presented method responds quite well for overlapping iodine seeds. In order to evaluate the precision of our algorithm the mean centroid error was calculated. The overall mean centroid error between ground-truth manual and automatic segmentations was 1.2 pixels, or 0.24mm when considering our pixel spacing of 0.2013mm. Due to the GUI used for the seed centroid extraction, manually segmented seeds could only be placed at the centers of the image pixels. Since the distance from the center of a pixel to one of its corner is equal to sqrt (0.5), we define this value as the pixel uncertainty associated with the manual segmentations. However, these results re-affirm the efficacy of the proposed algorithm.

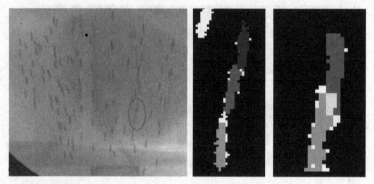

Fig. 5. Clinical example showing successful declustering in two- and three-seed clusters. (*Left*) the input X-ray image on the left is displayed, in red the three seed cluster is highlighted, in green the two-seed cluster. (*Right*) the detection of the seeds belonging to the three- and two- seed clusters respectively.

Clinical Implications: In reference to the D90 values—the minimum dose received by 90% of the prostate volume—Su et al. [9] state "*[t]he 95% confidence interval (CI) of estimated D90 values differ by less than 5% from the actual value when 95% or more seeds are detected, or approximately a 7 Gy difference in the D90 value for a prescription dose of 144 Gy.*" They concluded that accurate dose estimation can be achieved if 95% or more seeds are detected. Thus, our mean automatic detection rate of 98.7% surpasses clinical standards. Regarding segmentation, 84 seeds were not detected by our algorithm yielding an average of only 1.5 missed seeds per patient-image. Our results demonstrate a viable solution in the workflow of dynamic dosimetry (Figure 1) that ensures subsequent seed reconstruction in 3D and registration to TRUS data.

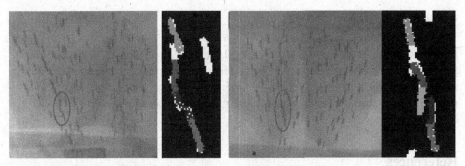

Fig. 6. Clinical examples depicting successful declustering of four-seed cluster on the left image and a <u>false</u> clustering of five-seeds in the right image

Drawbacks: 103 seeds were erroneously segmented, leading to a 1.7% false positive rate. This signifies that these were recognized by our algorithm as seeds; however they had no associated manual segmentation ground-truth. Here, it is observed that some identified clusters are not true clusters but a result from errors in the level set evolution (Figure 6-right), there is in fact two distinct clusters and not a five-seed cluster– a two- and three seed group).

Future Work: We aim at investigating filtering techniques, such as the homomorphic filter, that improves the original contrast of a newly acquired C-arm image during brachytherapy. We want to provide an initial image that optimizes the chances of the level set algorithm to lock onto seeds instead of *noisy* pixels. A natural extension of our algorithm is regarding the segmentation of other implants, such as ^{103}Pd or ^{137}Cs, which are used in prostate brachytherapy procedures. Also, color-coding the grayscale C-arm image which depicts individual or clustered seeds may facilitate seed correspondence between images for subsequent 3D reconstruction (Figure 7).

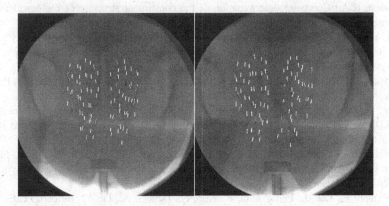

Fig. 7. C-arm imaged of the same patient showing clusters and individual seeds. A side benefit from colored segmentations: simplified seed correspondence.

5   Conclusions

In this work we have presented a practical technique to robustly segment prostate brachytherapy iodine implants thereby making an important contribution to both research and clinical practice. We have improved current state-of-art algorithms by proposing an n-seed declustering scheme for iodine seeds and positively validated the technique on patient datasets.

References

1. Siegel, R., Ward, E., Brawley, O., Jemal, A.: Cancer statistics. CA: Cancer J. Clin. 61(4), 212–236 (2011)
2. Nag, S., Ciezki, J.P., Cormack, R., Doggett, S., DeWyngaert, K., Edmundson, G.K., Stock, R.G., Stone, N.N., Yu, Y., Zelefsky, M.: Intraoperative planning and evaluation of permanent prostate brachy-therapy: report of the American brachytherapy society. International Journal of Radiation Oncology Biology Physics 51(5), 1422 (2001)
3. Lam, S., Marks, R.J., Cho, P.S.: Prostate brachytherapy seed segmentation using spoke transform. In: SPIE, vol. 4322(1), pp. 1490–1500 (2001)
4. Tubic, D., Zaccarin, A., Beaulieu, L., Pouliot, J.: Automated seed detection and three-dimensional reconstruction. i. seed localization from fluoroscopic images or radiographs. Medical Physics 28(11), 2272–2279 (2001)
5. Kuo, N., Deguet, A., Song, D.Y., Burdette, E.C., Prince, J.L., Lee, J.: Automatic segmentation of radiographic fiducial and seeds from x-ray images in prostate brachytherapy. Med. Eng. Phys. 34(1), 64–77 (2012)
6. Moult, E., Fichtinger, G., Morris, W., Salcudean, T., Dehghan, E., Fallavollita, P.: Segmentation of iodine brachytherapy implants in fluoroscopy. IJCARS 7(6), 871–879 (2012)
7. Li, C., Kao, C., Gore, J.C., Ding, Z.: Minimization of region-scalable fit- ting energy for image segmentation. IEEE Transactions on Image Processing 17, 1940–1949 (2008)
8. Kirsch, R.A.: Computer determination of the constituent structure of biological images. Computers and Biomedical Research 4, 315–328 (1971)
9. Su, Y., Davis, B., Herman, M., Manduca, A., Robb, R.: Examination of dosimetry accuracy as a func-tion of seed detection rate in permanent prostate brachytherapy. Med. Phys. 32, 30493056 (2001)
10. Hoskin, P., Coyle, C.: Radiotherapy in Practice - Brachytherapy. Radiotherapy in Practice Series. Oxford University Press (2011)
11. Lee, J., Labat, C., Jain, A.K., Song, D.Y., Burdette, C.E., Fichtinger, G., Prince, J.L.: REDMAPS: Reduced-Dimensionality Matching for Prostate Brachytherapy Seed Reconstruction. IEEE Transactions on Medical Imaging 30(1), 38–51 (2011)
12. Fallavollita, P., Karim Aghaloo, Z., Burdette, E.C., Song, D.Y., Abolmaesumi, P., Fichtinger, G.: Registration between ultrasound and fluoroscopy or CT in prostate brachytherapy. Medical Physics 37(6), 2749–2760 (2010)
13. Dehghan, E., Lee, J., Fallavollita, P., Kuo, N., Deguet, A., Le, Y., Burdette, C.E., Song, D.Y., Prince, J.L., Fichtinger, G.: Ultrasound–fluoroscopy registration for prostate brachytherapy dosimetry. Medical Image Analysis 16(7), 1347–1358 (2012)

Author Index